BE WELL!

BE WELL!

Jewish Health and Welfare in Glasgow, 1860–1914

Kenneth E. Collins

TUCKWELL PRESS

First published in Great Britain in 2001 by
Tuckwell Press
The Mill House
Phantassie
East Linton
East Lothian EH40 3DG

ISBN 1 86232 129 9

British Library Cataloguing in Publication Data
A catalogue record for this book is available
on request from the British Library

Typeset by Hewer Text Ltd, Edinburgh
Printed and bound by
Bell and Bain Ltd, Glasgow

Contents

Foreword

Kenneth Collins combines rare distinction in three quite different roles: as a doctor, a historian and a leader of the Glasgow Jewish community. In the present book he brings his unique tripartite expertise to tell the story of health issues as they affected Glasgow Jewry from the mid-Victorian period to the beginning of the First World War. Fascinating in its own right, it sheds light on a number of related issues – economic conditions in the largely immigrant community, the networks of self-help they created, and the entry of some of their own members into the medical profession, where they eventually achieved positions of great eminence. This is social history at its best, and has much to tell us about immigrant communities today.

The Jews who arrived in Scotland in the late nineteeth and early twentieth centuries were, for the most part, fleeing from persecution in Eastern Europe. In 1881 pogroms had broken out in more than a hundred Russian towns and cities, to be followed by the viciously anti-Semitic May Law of 1882. Millions of Jews fled to the West. Most of them were poor and faced huge difficulties in their new lands – learning a new language, adapting to new and strange culture, making a living and somehow piecing together the fragments of a shattered life. Not surprisingly, they suffered from poor housing and hygiene and the attendant problems of health. What they had – as Beatrice Webb noted in her study of London' poor Jews – was what economists today call 'social capital', strong families and communities, a collective ethos, an ancient but vigorous faith, and a deeply rooted sense of hope. Individually vulnerable, they gave one another strength. They founded *chevrot*, friendly societies, and *landsmanschaft* organisations, that eased some of the strains of dislocation and allowed them, in the course of one or two generations, to break free from the cycle of deprivation.

As Dr. Collins explains, their experiences were not easy. As today, there were many in Britain who opposed a relatively open immigration policy. They seized on health problems within the Jewish community to argue for more restrictive entry, which eventually came in the form of the 1905 Aliens Act. There were tensions between the new arrivals and the more established Jewish families. There was also a deep ambivalence about some of the evangelical Christian groups who offered help but at the same time sought to convert the newcomers to their faith. It is a story full of drama – the human drama that occurs whenever a group is forced to leave one country for another. It is never easy. There are always conflicts of pain and adjustment. In the end, though, this is a story of hope.

The Jews who came to Glasgow never lost their sense of gratitude to the place that had given them refuge. High among their priorities was a desire to give back, to contribute, which they did in many ways over the years. They remembered the words of the prophet Jeremiah, engraved for millennia on the Jewish heart: 'Seek the peace and prosperity of the city to which I have carried you and pray to the Lord for it, because its welfare will be your welfare'. That twin vocation of remaining true to one's faith while bringing a blessing to the larger society has been the Jewish way since the days of Abraham and Sarah. It is a long and ancient story, of which the Glasgow Jewish community has been a distinguished chapter.

'Remember the days of old,' said Moses in one of the last speeches of his life. 'Consider the generations long past; ask your father to recount it and your elders to tell the tale.' Remembering, in Judaism, is a religious duty, because memory is the moral tutor of mankind. The story of the past, its achievements and shortcomings, its errors and successes, is our best guide as we face the future. We are indebted to Kenneth Collins for this splendid study of a time of upheaval for both Scots and Jews. From it, both communities emerged with great credit, and in so doing taught us an important lesson: the non-zero-sumness of human goodness. Glasgow gave much to its Jews, and the Jewish community gave much to Glasgow. Both gained; both grew; and between them developed a friendship and mutual respect which remains strong today and I pray will continue long into the future.

Chief Rabbi Professor Jonathan Sacks
Erev Shabbat Nachamu 5761
3rd August 2001

Illustrations

Abbreviations

GEI	Glasgow Eye Infirmary
GGHB	Greater Glasgow Health Board
GHC	Glasgow Hebrew Congregation
GJHFSVA	Glasgow Jewish Hospital Fund and Sick Visiting Association
LJBG	London Jewish Board of Guardians
SJAC	Scottish Jewish Archives Centre
US	United Synagogue

The publishers acknowledge subsidy from the Guthrie Trust of the Scottish Society for the History of Medicine, the Walton Foundation, the Greater Glasgow Health Board Ethnic Health Fund and the Scottish Jewish Archives Centre towards the publication of this volume.

Acknowledgements

This book has taken about ten years to write sandwiched between the busy life of a general medical practitioner and the engrossing task of leadership in the Glasgow Jewish community. My history of the Jews in Glasgow, *Second City Jewry: the Jews of Glasgow in the Age of Expansion 1790–1919*, was published in 1990 and introduced many health and welfare related topics. At my first International Congress on the History of Medicine in Antwerp in 1990, the 33rd Congress, I presented a paper on 'The Jews of Glasgow: Aspects of Health and Welfare 1790-1920'. I returned to the theme at the 35th International Congress in Kos in 1996 with a paper on 'Immigrant mental health in Glasgow: the Jewish Experience' and at the 36th International Congress in Tunis in 1998 with a paper on 'Trachoma and the Alien Immigrant in Glasgow'. The material on the Jews in medicine in Glasgow is condensed from two presentations. The first, on the Levenston family, entitled 'Medical Orthodoxy and Reform: Differing Medical Practices in a Glasgow Jewish Victorian family', was made to the 34th International Congress on the History of Medicine in Glasgow in 1994 and published in *Korot: the Israel Journal of Medicine and Science* in 1995. The second presentation, on 'Asher Asher MD: Victorian Physician and Medical Reformer', was made at a Conference on 'Medical Professionals: Identities, Interests and Ideology' under the auspices of the Society for the Social History of Medicine in Glasgow in July 1999.

As a Research Associate at the Wellcome Unit for the History of Medicine at the University of Glasgow I have benefited from the guidance and support of Dr. Marguerite Dupree and Dr. Malcolm Nicholson and have welcomed the opportunity to present some early findings at Unit seminars. The Scottish Jewish Archives Centre, at the Garnethill Synagogue in Glasgow, is a rich resource for the study of the Jewish communities of Scotland and I am grateful to its Director, Harvey Kaplan, and my Co-chairman, Dr. Jack E Miller, for their friendship and co-operation.

I would also like to express my thanks to the following individuals and institutions:

Alistair Tough and Karl Magee, Archivists, Greater Glasgow Health Board

Morag Williams, Archivist, Dumfries and Galloway Health Board

Dr. Louise Yeoman, Division of Manuscripts, National Library of Scotland, Edinburgh

Howard Markel, Director, Historical Center for the Health Sciences, University of Michigan

Charles Tucker, Record Keeper, London Beth Din

Glasgow Room and Departments of Health, Religion and Philosophy, and History at the Mitchell Library, Glasgow

London Metropolitan Archives

National Archives of Scotland, Edinburgh

Hartley Library, University of Southampton

Library, London School of Jewish Studies

Jewish Care, London

Derek and Joan Anderson, of London, for sharing their family knowledge about Asher Asher

Gerald Levenston of Toronto, Ontario and his son Michael Levenston of Vancouver, British Columbia, for supplying a copy of (Solomon) Alexander Levenston's pharmacopeia, details of Joseph Levenston's correspondence and for filling in some of the missing details in the complex family tree.

This book has been produced on my now ancient Amstrad PCW8512, which has survived, more or less, to see this work concluded. My thanks go to Michael Simpson for transferring the material to a more modern PC format. My thanks to my mother, Dr. Hetty Collins, and to my children, Eve and Josh; Tamar, Daniel and Adi; Rachel and David for their encouragement. Finally, as ever I am grateful to my wife Irene who has not only helped with retrieving material for me but has cheerfully attended the Congresses where some of this material was first presented. Without her none of this would have been possible.

Introduction

'The notoriety which Glasgow has gained over the past years is nowhere more evident than in the field of health and health care. Experts have come to Glasgow to be shocked. They have rarely been disappointed.'
Olive Checkland and Margaret Lamb, eds., *Health Care as Social History: the Glasgow Case* (Aberdeen,1982), p.6

'Among Jews in Eastern Europe the parting greeting was not the meaningless 'cheerio' or 'goodbye' or even 'au revoir' but *zei gezunt* (be well) . . . The expression *zei gezunt* represents not merely a benign wish, but is tantamount almost to a positive commandment.'
Chaim Bermant, *The Jews* (London, 1978), paperback edition, pp.137–138

This is the story of health issues in a new immigrant community in Glasgow around the turn of the twentieth century and examines the issues of ethnicity and religion in the provision of health and welfare. The story links the Jewish community of Glasgow during the main immigrant period, from 1860–1914, a growing community struggling to adapt to its new environment and a city possessing both a remarkable medical infrastructure and some of the worst health statistics in Britain. It aims to examine the areas, related to welfare and health, in which the Jews of Glasgow interacted with the host society as well as the coping strategies they employed to help their integration. The story will show difficulties as well as successes and highlights the problems faced by a group with different origins, language, religion and customs from the society in which they settled. While Scotland in general, and Glasgow in particular, has always been proud of its relationship with its Jewish community, aspects of that relationship produced strains which have not wholly disappeared.

Above all it tells of a single Jewish community, and its concerns with health and welfare, while it grappled with the problems of settlement and integration. Glasgow's Jews settled in a city that already had an infrastructure for health and education, and statutory provision was always a useful supplement to communal endeavours. Without it the impressive array of community facilities would not have succeeded.[1]

The Jews of Glasgow brought the best elements of the *shtetl* with them to Glasgow, in the form of a society adapted to self-help and a propensity to develop communal structures for every possible area of perceived welfare, educational, religious or social need. They also had the advantage that, whenever they arrived in the city, they found that the Jews already settled in Glasgow had established a network of institutions which facilitated their integration while preserving their distinct heritage. These were based around the Garnethill Synagogue, founded in 1879, but successor to previous synagogues dating back to 1823.

The small size of the Jewish community in Glasgow, which even at its peak never exceeded 15,000, prevented the formation of larger Jewish institutions, like a hospital, and delayed the successful establishment of a Jewish Old Age Home until the end of the first half of the twentieth century. Likewise, the small size of the more integrated and assimilated community, based at the Garnethill Synagogue, meant that the size of the elite was too small to dominate the relatively large influx which later overwhelmed it.[2] Garnethill's financial and numerical weakness prejudiced its chances of establishing true control over developments in the new immigrant areas around the Gorbals, south of the River Clyde.

The immigrant period has been a fruitful area of study for Jewish historians, and the role of the London Jewish elite in its philanthropic relationship with the poor newcomers has been the subject of much debate, often based on class lines.[3] The Garnethill elite was able to maintain some control of communal institutions until well into the twentieth century. Even within the Garnethill Synagogue itself, the system of elected seat-holders, in operation during the main period of immigration, ensured that communal power was concentrated in relatively few hands. However, the Glasgow experience was of a Jewish leadership, in a position of authority because of earlier arrival in the city, striking a balance between community discipline and immigrant innovation. That is not to say that conflict between the groups north and south of the River Clyde did not exist, and as we shall see that conflict could be expressed in the most graphic of terms. Nevertheless, Garnethill knew its obligations, as well as its limitations, and the result, from the entire community, was a welfare network acknowledged to be ahead of its time.

Garnethill had a long involvement in the Yiddish language Talmud Torah elementary educational classes, founded in the Gorbals in 1895, and in a series of synagogue unions with the Gorbals synagogues and *chevras*. These activities showed the extraordinary lengths to which they were prepared to go to maintain links with Gorbals Jewry, and to tolerate its ways. The Glasgow United Synagogue broke up in 1906 amid recriminations over such issues as the management of *shechita* and pauper funerals at a time when the increasing number of synagogues in the Gorbals made it impossible for one synagogue, no matter how prestigious, to dominate all the others. However, there persisted a feeling in the Gorbals that the Garnethill leadership had greater skills, and there was undoubtedly a sense of awe and reverence in the Gorbals for the Garnethill achievements.[4]

The Glasgow Jewish Board of Guardians maintained its austere image and organisational unity, despite the formation of a plethora of small, poorly funded charitable bodies in the Gorbals, and retained its base at Garnethill until 1912. By this time control of the institutions of Glasgow Jewry was passing to the new community in the Gorbals, and the Garnethill-based leadership of the Board of Guardians could no longer ignore calls for a welfare centre in the heart of the community it was serving. While the Board of Guardians tried to maintain a coherent, community-wide welfare strategy, it had neither the resources nor the control of the small Gorbals welfare bodies to make such a strategy successful.

The Board struggled to meets its obligations to the Jewish poor even with the growth of the friendly societies which provided welfare and medical benefits that its members felt that they had earned.

The formation of the Glasgow Jewish Representative Council in 1914, with Joseph Hallside, a Gorbals tailor, as its President, illustrated the passage of power from Garnethill, and its widely admired patrician leader Michael Simons. The fledgling Council lacked the expertise of the Garnethill leadership while Garnethill-based bodies, like the Jewish Literary Society and the Jewish Board of Guardians, did not affiliate to the Council at first. However, when the community had to approach local or national government bodies, the continuing leading role of the Garnethill Synagogue was recognised. There might be the formation of joint delegations of Synagogue and Council or even the setting up of joint structures under the Garnethill leadership.[5] In London, the Jewish Board of Guardians was involved in a systematic mass repatriation policy that returned over 50,000 Jews to Eastern Europe between 1882 and 1914. While some family re-unions were arranged by the Glasgow Jewish Board of Guardians, this was on a deliberately small scale, as a 'last resort' and with the full consent of those involved.[6]

The Glasgow, proudly described as the 'Second City' of the British Empire, that the Jewish newcomers had settled in was a city of power, prestige and poverty. Its manufacturing base had attracted a wide variety of immigrants to work in its industries or in the many associated commercial activities which grew rapidly in the prosperous manufacturing sector. Jews quickly found work in tailoring, cigarette making or peddling, some moving on to open their own shops, factories and warehouses as their businesses succeeded. The new arrivals saw their goals as personal economic stability, combined with the establishment of the conditions for an educational base from which their children could readily advance. Their social and economic mobility needed little encouragement.[7] One way out of the ghetto trades was education. The Jewish community was quick to take advantage of the schooling available and Jews started to enter university from the middle of the nineteenth century. By the start of the First World War there were the first signs of a developing professional class as the immigrants' sons entered medicine. The struggle for health and wellbeing had its parallel in the struggle to enter the medical profession.

There was, however, another side to Glasgow life. Its sweated workshops and festering slum properties bred generations of workers, and their families, with a propensity to health problems. Jewish community leaders were keen to point out the nature of Jewish self-reliance and their supportive communal structure and they claimed that Jewish health and housing conditions were better than those of their neighbours. Thus, the Jewish community were less affected by many of the acute infections, such as typhoid and typhus, which were prevalent in Glasgow. Yet, there were still some acknowledged persistent Jewish health problems such as a particularly chronic problem with tuberculosis, which lasted at least until the end of the First World War.

Despite the problems of poverty, the new Jewish immigrants to Glasgow scored well on health indices. Infant mortality was significantly lower among the Jews of Glasgow than that of their neighbours at a time when the Jewish birth rate was higher. A study of the diets of Glasgow families carried out during 1911–1912 showed a better understanding of nutrition in the Jewish households in the Gorbals, and there was a lower incidence of rickets.

With trachoma, the Glasgow Medical Officer of Health felt that he had identified a disease, prevalent in Jewish aliens, which could be controlled by restrictions on immigration. Though the evidence for this was weak, it was politically more acceptable to call for alien immigration control on medical, rather than racial, grounds. Because of its peculiar visibility, opponents of Jewish immigration, often racially motivated, claimed that trachoma represented the dangerous infectious nature of the alien Jew with his contagious eye disease. Trachoma was one of the most common causes for refusal of entry in the first years after the passage of the Aliens Act

(1905) but its incidence did not match the fears expressed by the opponents of Jewish immigration.

Jews had a variety of contacts with the hospitals. There were negotiations with the Victoria Infirmary over the provision of kosher food, a request to which the hospital was reluctant to accede in case there were other requests for exemption from the regular meals. For Jewish patients, the greatest problems were faced by those with mental illness, who were admitted into the lunatic asylums of Glasgow from the 1890s. By using the hospital records we can see contemporary attitudes to Jewish patients and their illnesses. Jewish patients faced problems related to the unfamiliar surroundings, such as with food and language, compounded by the added difficulties related to delusional illness. There was a reluctance to enter the psychiatric hospital, or indeed the Poorhouse, partly due to the supportive Jewish network in the Gorbals, but also because of the fear of unfamiliar institutions where Jewish festivals and the dietary laws would not be observed.

While, in general, Jews integrated well into their new surroundings, the relationship with the Christian majority was marred by the presence in the Gorbals of groups of evangelical missionaries who aimed to 'win the Jews for Christ' by offering medical, social and welfare benefits. At an official level, the various Christian churches were seen as supportive of the Jewish community in the issues that concerned them. There was Christian support for the Jewish plight in Russia, and for exemptions from Sunday trading laws for those observing the Jewish Sabbath.[8] On the street, however, the Christian churches seemed much less friendly. Jews saw the missionary effort as questioning the legitimacy of their faith, and the conflict between the mission hall and the Jewish community soured Jewish-Christian relations for many decades.

Glasgow Jewry emerged stronger, and more self-reliant, from its struggle for health in the immigrant period. The combination of communal philanthropy, Christian missionary competition and community-based societies produced a healthier and stronger community, with pride in its achievements, which served as an example to newer immigrant groups.

References

1 Eugene C Black, *The Social Politics of Anglo-Jewry 1880–1920* (Oxford, 1988), pp.3–4.
2 Kenneth Collins, *Second City Jewry: the Jews of Glasgow in the Age of Expansion 1790–1919* (Glasgow, 1990), p.219.
3 Mordechai Rozin, *The Rich and the Poor: Jewish Philanthropy and Social Control in Nineteenth-Century London* (Brighton, 1999), pp.5–6.
4 Isaac Hirshow, Speech on occasion of his 25th anniversary as *Chazan* of the Garnethill Hebrew Congregation, 3/12/1950. SJAC.
5 *Jewish Chronicle*, 11/9/1914.
6 *Jewish Chronicle*, 15/12/1905.
7 Lloyd P Gartner, 'Eastern European Jewish Immigrants in England: a quarter-century's view', *Jewish Historical Studies*, Vol. XXXIX (1982–1986), pp.297–310.
8 *Jewish Chronicle*, 22/6/1906.

CHAPTER ONE

The Origins of Glasgow Jewry

'. . . the appearance of so many setting aside the best evidence of the most blessed testimony is humbling and distressing.'
Rev. James Brown, commenting on the opening of the George Street Synagogue, 1858, *The Religious Denominations of Glasgow*, Volume 1 (Glasgow, 1860)

While individual Jews have been living and working in Glasgow since the end of the eighteenth century, the growth in Glasgow's Jewish community remained slow for many years, only increasing substantially in the last years of the nineteenth century and the first years of the twentieth. The Glasgow Hebrew Congregation was established in 1823, with a small synagogue in two rooms of a first-floor flat at 43 High Street, near the Trongate in the city centre. By 1831, when a census was taken of the Jewish citizens of Glasgow, the community numbered thirty-one souls about half of whom had been born in England, with many of the others immigrants from Poland, Germany and Holland.[1] These thirty-one Jews formed a tiny minority of the 200,000 inhabitants of Glasgow, whose population was growing considerably under the pressures of industrial and commercial development.

Glasgow became the economic magnet that drew immigrants from many sources, from within Scotland and beyond, transforming the city from a small university town to one of the great Victorian industrial centres. By the end of the nineteenth century Glasgow styled itself the 'Second City' of the British Empire, exceeded in size and trade only by London. The economy of Scotland had been developing rapidly during the nineteenth and twentieth centuries. This development was accompanied by a major population shift, especially from the Highlands, but also from other rural areas to the towns and cities of the Scottish Lowlands. During this time Scotland had the fastest rate of urbanisation of any European country and its urban population was, proportionally, only exceeded by that of England and Wales.[2]

The first Jewish community to be established in Scotland was in Edinburgh in 1816. There had been individual Jews in Edinburgh from the seventeenth century, and while the number of Jews in Glasgow and Edinburgh remained small during the first half of the nineteenth century, it was Glasgow's explosive Victorian industrial and commercial growth which attracted so many incomers. The first Jews in Glasgow were, in the main, business merchants taking advantage of the commercial opportunities offered by the thriving city and its new entrepreneurial class. By the middle of the nineteenth century agents of shipping and textile companies from Hamburg, who set up business in Dundee and Glasgow from 1840 to purchase cheap linens and packing cloths, were augmenting Glasgow Jewry.[3] In 1842, Glasgow Jewry, still numbering less than 200 souls, suffered major communal dissension over the opening of a synagogue at the Andersonian University. As the building contained a medical school, where anatomical studies and dissection took place, a minority contended that it was against Jewish principles to hold services in such a place. For the next few years the small community organised two sets of services, of Hebrew classes and of welfare facilities. The split was only healed when a new synagogue in Howard Street was opened in 1849.

One of Glasgow's strengths appeared to be a ready acceptance of people of ability without regard to their origins. The growing middle classes formed the market for the Jewish furriers, jewellers, glue and quill merchants, agents and warehousemen who played an increasing role in the life of the city. Obviously not all businesses were successful and there are records of bankruptcies of various Jewish businesses, in such fields as jewellery, oilcloths and wines and spirits during the 1850s.[4]

Increasing membership and a growing prosperity were the catalysts for a major expansion of Jewish facilities with a new synagogue in George Street opening in 1858. With about 200 seats this new development accommodated four times as many worshippers and indicated a new phase in the life of Glasgow Jewry. Some £30 of the first £300 raised for the building came from Christian friends, and the wider community was well represented at the ceremonies marking the opening of the synagogue.[5] The Jewish leadership intended that their new synagogue would set the seal on their community's acceptance as an integral part of the life of the growing city. It was important that they had a building as a place of worship that was felt to be worthy of their status. The *Glasgow Herald,* who commented favourably on Rev. Dr. Mayer's sermon, 'in English, with a foreign accent', covered the opening ceremony.[6] Another Christian visitor to the ceremony was the Rev. James Brown who commented positively on the Jews of Glasgow as 'moral, industrious, educated, and some of them wealthy, and they are united in their obedience to the Law of Moses'. However, his comments also included the view that 'the appearance of so many setting aside the best evidence of the most blessed testimony is humbling and distressing'.[7]

The relationship between Christians and Jews in Glasgow was relatively harmonious from the earliest years. The first Jewish burial ground, opened in 1831, was a small Jewish section in the prestigious new Glasgow Necropolis, laid out in the fashion of the Père la Chaise Cemetery in Paris.[8] The sale of this ground to the Jewish community, for 100 guineas, enough for fifty-one interments, indicates the success of the Jewish newcomers and their acceptance into the life of the city. Not all the inhabitants of the city shared the same warm sentiments. Some Christian clergymen, like the Rev. James Brown, found it difficult to accept the presence of a Jewish community in a city that had no previous history of non-Christian worship. As we shall see, Scottish Presbyterian messianism led to the formation of the first Scottish society for mission to the Jews in 1838 when the Jewish presence in both Glasgow and Edinburgh, though small, was clearly established.[9] The relationship between Jews and Christians in Glasgow was to maintain two clear components. On one side there were those who showed great favour to the Jewish community and provided practical help in times of real need, such as during the pogroms in Russia, while others maintained a purely missionary intent and provided services and sermons which aimed, ultimately, to entice the Jews from their faith.[10]

The first signs of what eventually developed into a major transmigration route from Eastern Europe to North America, passing through Glasgow, can be discerned from the 1860s.[11] Jews were being attracted to Britain by unsettled conditions, both political and economic, in Central and Eastern Europe with a majority coming from Russia and Poland, and the balance from Germany and Holland. This balance was reflected in Glasgow where the predominant Jewish element in the city on the eve of the mass immigration was Russian and Polish.

This growth during the 1860s and 1870s led to further demands for a larger synagogue that could house all the Jews of the growing city. However, by this time the geographical base of the community was enlarging. The Jews no longer formed a small compact group in the streets around the city centre. Some of the more prosperous were moving to the new townhouses stretching westwards along Bath Street, though a significant and poorer group were still to be found in the streets around the city centre near the George Street Synagogue. At the same time a new industrial group was forming in the Gorbals just to the south of the River Clyde.

Growth and Development

The community's growth was suddenly reinforced during the 1870s by the arrival of a large group of tailors, mostly from London, who had been recruited by the Glasgow firm of Arthur and Company, or more probably by a Jewish employee within the company, to introduce new methods of clothing production to Glasgow.[12] Quickly, some of these tailors established their own companies, whether in tailoring or in other fields. Settling mainly in the Gorbals, they found the short distance across the river to George Street little problem. However, when the growth in the community necessitated the building of a new synagogue, the site chosen was in Garnet Street, at the western end of the city centre. This was really suitable only for those in the older-established community.

The opposition to the new synagogue site, distant as it was from the homes of the poorest sections of the community, was easily defeated at a meeting of the voting members and seat-holders of the George Street Synagogue in November 1875.[13] Thus, a new and imposing synagogue was eventually erected at Garnethill, opening in September 1879. This building cost the substantial sum of £13,000, though incurring debts which took a generation to pay off. Again, it was felt that the building of an imposing place of worship with decorous services would raise the status of the Jewish community in the wider society.[14] During the building, when the congregation was briefly homeless, a decision was made to look for premises, which could be used for Hebrew Classes in a more central part of town, suitable for children from south of the river. It was clear that with Jewish settlement proceeding westwards from the city centre, as well as forming south of the river, the time when these two factors would necessitate the formation of two distinct Jewish centres could not be delayed indefinitely. By the time of the 1891 Census about half of Glasgow Jewry were living in or around the Gorbals area while the original area of Jewish settlement, to the east and south of George Square, saw its numbers depleted as the more prosperous members of the community moved westwards, around the area of the new Garnethill Synagogue. By the end of the nineteenth century Glasgow Jewry was overwhelmingly centred south of the river.

There were a number of areas of potential conflict, both religious and organisational, between the larger group around the new Garnethill Synagogue and the smaller group of poorer newcomers south of the river in the Gorbals. The voting power of the synagogue was vested in the hands of the older membership.[15] Voting rights belonged only to seat-holders, a position attained only by election, by existing seat-holders, from among the regular membership. The membership fee of £3 meant that only the best paid of Jewish workers would have been able to afford to become seat-holders. This concentrated power, and decision-making, in the hands of a relatively small number of men and built up frustrations in the more religious newcomers who were denied a say in the synagogue affairs on financial grounds. It was hardly surprising that the opening of the new synagogue at Garnethill precipitated the establishment of the first Jewish *chevra* in the Gorbals.[16]

Religious differences were also apparent. The more accultured Garnethill community had long ceased to hold services during the week. They had made some modifications to the service, such as having a mixed choir and scrapping the priestly blessing on festival days. For Gorbals Jewry the synagogue was a male preserve, with services three times daily, often accompanied by study of religious literature and, in the early days, little thought either for style or decorum. The established leadership looked on this development with dismay. As Williams has pointed out, the more accultured leadership would have felt threatened by the semi-autonomy of the *chevra*, regarding its ethos as unacceptable and its cultural isolation as dangerous.[17] One letter writer from Glasgow noted in the *Jewish Chronicle* that '. . . there was a need to anglicise the community'[18] while another Glasgow correspondent, fearing the damage that an undisciplined organisation might do to community relations, commented that 'a *shul* with a dignified service will do a vast deal more to raise Judaism in our neighbours' esteem than our upright and honourable (Jewish) behaviour'.[19]

However, Garnethill recognised the need to keep some degree of control over the new community, and this schism was not allowed to sever relationships north and south of the river. A series of synagogue unions were put into force over the next twenty years in which the Garnethill Synagogue worked relentlessly to exert some form of authority over the institutions of the newcomers in the Gorbals.[20] At first this involved a 'take over' of the *chevra,* with Gorbals residents who were also Garnethill seat-holders in a position of leadership.[21] There then followed a simple arrangement whereby the main Gorbals synagogue functioned as a subsidiary branch synagogue of Garnethill. With further communal growth and an expansion in the number of Gorbals synagogues this arrangement had to change. Accordingly, in 1898 the United Synagogue of Glasgow was established as a loose federation of independent synagogues. The organisational arrangements ensured that the Garnethill leadership maintained control of the new body and continued to exercise authority through the eight years, from 1898 to 1906, that the United Synagogue remained in existence.

The United Synagogue itself collapsed in 1906 after major disagreements on a number of key issues involving the provision of kosher meat and problems related to the responsibility for payment of pauper funerals.[22] With the prevalence of infectious diseases in the poorest sections of the community, there was a high death rate amongst children, as well as adults, creating a communal financial burden beyond the resources of the synagogues and welfare bodies. The only solvent communal body capable of meeting these costs were the *shechita* bodies, which supplied kosher meat and derived an income from its sale. A further source of friction between Garnethill and Gorbals was the presence, in the Gorbals, of a Garnethill licensed kosher poultry yard which, it was claimed, took money from the Gorbals poor to subsidise the Garnethill Synagogue mortgage.[23]

Following the collapse of the United Synagogue, a number of attempts were made to provide Jewish leadership in a united, Glasgow-wide body. Some of these bodies were charitable, educational and religious. Some, like the Jewish Communal Council set up in 1907, had representative functions but only dealt with Gorbals issues. A Glasgow Jewish Representative Council, capable of acting on behalf of all the Jewish organisations in Glasgow, was not established until 1914, in the wake of the community-wide protests related to the Mendel Beilis blood libel trial in Kiev.[24] However, even after the setting up of the Glasgow Jewish Representative Council, the strength and influence of the Garnethill Synagogue, some of whose associated institutions were deliberately slow to affiliate to the Council, ensured that in matters of importance the Council and Garnethill had to work together. Garnethill was thus more than just *primus inter pares.*

Transmigration

As we have seen, there were Jews passing through Glasgow on the transmigration route from the 1860s, and the beginnings of the Gorbals Jewish community can be discerned from the 1870s. Thus it is not surprising that the geographical origins of the immigrants after 1880 were not so different from arrivals before that date. Indeed it was estimated in 1881 that three-quarters of Glasgow Jewry were of Russian and Polish origin with Jews from Germany and Holland forming a comparatively small part.[25]

The events of 1881 and 1882 in Russia, with the passage of the May Laws, and the evidence of clear, government-led hostility to the Jews, gave a sense of urgency to a population already demoralised by poverty, overcrowding and unemployment. By 1882 much of Eastern Europe was on the move. While millions were to seek the shores of the New World, about 120,000 Jews arrived in Britain between 1882 and 1914. However, the early flood of Jewish immigration did not come to Glasgow, unlike London and Manchester where the flow of Jews began in the crisis days of 1882. In fact, only about 1,000 Jews arrived in Glasgow during the 1880s and the main growth in the Glasgow Jewish community only came with further restrictions in Russia, enforced in 1891.[26] Thus, the health and welfare issues thrown up by the new immigration did not become apparent until the last years of the nineteenth century and the first years of the twentieth century.

Despite the relatively small immigration in the early 1880s, events in Russia had a resonance in Glasgow. On February 2nd 1882, on the day following the great Mansion House meeting in London, a crowd of 3,000 gathered at the St. Andrew's Hall in Glasgow to hear protests about the notorious May Laws, and the pogroms which followed.[27] The Lord Provost, John Ure, provided leadership for the meeting but there was support too from the major churches including the Moderator of the Glasgow Presbytery of the Church of Scotland and Archbishop Eyre of the Roman

Catholic Church. This church support for Jewish suffering was a recurring theme as the Jewish tragedy in Russia unfolded over subsequent decades.

By 1891, immigration patterns were clearer as the 'Russian and Polish' element predominated. In fact, the bulk of the new Jewish immigrants to Glasgow derived from the Russian-ruled Baltic areas, particularly from Lithuania. The proximity of Lithuanian Jewry to the shipping and travel routes to Western and Central Europe and North America certainly made emigration easier at this time of stress and they increasingly formed a major element in western Jewish communities. Nevertheless, Glasgow's industrial expansion had made it a major centre of internal migration within Britain. In addition, records of some of the arrivals in Scotland show a wider distribution than from Lithuania alone, although this remained the most significant part of the make-up of Glasgow Jewry.

A substantial number of the children living in Glasgow in 1891 were born in various towns and cities in England. This shows the ease with which the Jewish population travelled round the immigrant areas of the country seeking employment. A few of the children had been born in Scotland outside Glasgow, usually Edinburgh but also Dundee, where a Jewish community had been founded in 1874, and Aberdeen, where a community was organised in 1893.[28] The presence of many children in a family could be an inhibiting factor in the decision to leave Eastern Europe. While a substantial number of couples had their first two children born abroad, the figures drop sharply for larger families. The prospects of travelling with a large number of children would have been daunting and might only be contemplated if the children were of an age to be earning themselves. The proportion of Jewish pupils in the Gorbals Primary School increased from 10% in 1890 (59 out of 570) to almost half (199 out of 402) just ten years later.[29]

The United States, popularly known as *di goldene medine*, the land where the streets were 'paved with gold', was the ultimate destination for most Jewish migrants. However, Glasgow became a suitable point for direct travel from Eastern Europe to the United

States when a properly organised transmigration route through the city commenced in 1886. This route was used by the Anchor Line, taking Scandinavians, as well as Jews from Eastern Europe, to America. The late start for this development explains the slower growth of Glasgow Jewry during the 1880s as Jewish workers had to be attracted to the city by better prospects than were available in any of the major English cities. Nevertheless, there was now scope to take advantage of Glasgow's position as a commercial and shipping centre.

The transmigrant route to America across Scotland was not just an alternative to the direct Atlantic crossing from Libau or Hamburg. Soon, a number of Scottish shipping companies were in competition with the English route, which led across the North Sea to Hull, then by rail to Liverpool. More than a million Jews travelled across England on this route on their way to North America.[30] Not all these travellers actually reached Liverpool as many dropped out at the various Jewish communities that grew up in the towns along the Hull-Liverpool railway line.

Though the numbers passing through Scotland were only a small proportion of the passengers on the Hull to Liverpool route, it still proved lucrative for the shipping companies and financially competitive for the travellers. After crossing the North Sea to Dundee or Leith there followed a train ride either to Glasgow, to catch the steamer to America from the Broomielaw, in the heart of Glasgow, or to the port of Greenock on the Firth of Clyde. Greenock's position as the last point on the Scottish transmigration route led to the establishment of a small Jewish community in about 1891.[31] In Glasgow too, the synagogue authorities at Garnethill took steps to ensure that the needs of these travellers were being met. The transmigration process was fraught with dangers. Thieves and tricksters could be found at all stages of the journey to rob the unsuspecting wayfarers, and it was the Jewish community itself, rather than the ports or the police, which cleaned up the British docks.[32]

However, it was some years before significant numbers of these travellers began to 'drop out' in Glasgow, though they still intended to cross the Atlantic at a later date. Some travellers dropped out of necessity, having expended all their savings on the first stages of their journey. Many transmigrants, however, paid for the whole journey from Eastern Europe to America in advance, as this would have been cheaper than for a two-stage journey via Glasgow. In Glasgow there was the opportunity to learn English, adapt to the new ways in business and make contacts in the local community, knowing that there was the possibility of further opportunities to the west if things did not work out. So the Jewish community gradually increased as more newcomers were attracted by the presence of relatives or *landsleit* in the city who could provide work or smooth the process of integration.

The increase in the community, and in British Jewry as a whole, followed further developments in Russia. In 1890 there were persistent reports from Russia that further anti-Jewish measures were being prepared, and in the following year the storm broke. Jews living in cities, such as Moscow, which lay outside the Pale of Settlement, were summarily expelled, and in addition to anti-Semitic administrative edicts came further terror and violence in many other parts of the country. Jewry was on the move westwards. There is still debate about the relative importance of economic or political factors in swelling the emigration from Russia. It is clear from contemporary evidence that physical persecution played a part in the decision to emigrate. It is also clear that economic conditions in Eastern Europe were desperate. However, Jews mostly emigrated from areas furthest from the pogroms, especially from the Baltic provinces, but also from Galicia in southern Poland, then under a relatively benign Austrian rule, as well as from Rumania.

Travelling conditions for the transmigrants, whose financial resources had been exhausted in the costs of their tickets, were horrendous. In July 1891 a group of transmigrants arriving in Leith were in a 'wretched state' and were supplied with food by the Jewish community in Edinburgh before they were able to travel to Glasgow.[33] Soon two boatloads of Jewish refugees were arriving in Leith every week.[34] Readers of the *Scotsman* raised £200 to help pay for the costs of looking after these Jewish refugees as they crossed Scotland. A further group of fifty-three Jews travelling across Scotland in October of that year were reported as being barely able to fast on *Yom Kippur*, after a rough North Sea crossing, and one of their number had to be hospitalised in Leith.[35]

Many of the travellers arriving in Scotland had desperate tales to tell. In August 1891 the arrivals included a widow with five children who had been summarily evicted from the inn she had run in a small village near Odessa, and many others who had been uprooted from their homes and livelihoods. Other stories were equally heartrending. One Jewish refugee en route in Leith recounted that he was '. . . one of a company of sixty who tried to cross the frontier. They endeavoured to bribe the sentries with £1.50 each. The bribe was taken but forty-six were captured and thrown back into prison, some to be exiled to Siberia and the rest, at great risk, escaped'.[36] By September 1891, it was clear that more Jews were stopping their journey in Glasgow, and it was noted that 'a large influx of destitute immigrants are settling in the city where conditions are deplorable'.[37]

By the end of the nineteenth, and early in the twentieth century, the majority of those beginning their sea voyage on their way to America from Glasgow or Greenock were Jewish. The figures varied considerably from year to year but numbers were increasing substantially with over 10,500 travellers of varying backgrounds making the crossing in 1893, and though numbers fell to just over 1,500 in 1898 they increased again to over 6,000 in 1902 and 1903.[38] The number of travellers, and their poverty and health, posed a strain for the communities they passed through, with Edinburgh in particular claiming that proportionately they had done more for the refugees than any other local community.[39]

Community Growth

Glasgow Jewry's growth continued in the pre-War period. Although the level of immigration was decreasing, the migration of a relatively youthful population helped stimulate natural increase. Thus, while there was significant onward emigration, especially to North America, the community was still expanding. During the first years of the century about 3,000 transmigrants passed through Glasgow, of whom about one third were Jewish, but the total number of transmigrants rose substantially to 19,828 in 1908, mostly travelling on the Anchor Line. About 4,200 were classified as Jewish but many, and probably most, of the additional 5,700 described as being Polish and Russian were also Jewish. This substantial increase in transmigrants continued until the First World War.[40] Besides these arrivals many other Jews were encouraged to come to Glasgow by the Jewish Dispersion Committee, which sought to ease the congestion in the Jewish areas of the East End of London.[41]

According to contemporary estimates in 1898 and 1902 the size of the community had grown to between 6,500 and 8,000 compared to only about 2,000 a decade earlier. Records of births, or at least circumcisions, marriages and deaths were well maintained by the Glasgow Hebrew Congregation and subsequently for the United Synagogue. However, this will not include members of the smaller groups outwith the main synagogues. In 1899 there were about 50 deaths each year but this figure rose to between 90 and 100 a few years later.[42] The majority of the deaths were stillbirths and children under the age of 16 years. There were more than 250 Jewish births in Glasgow in 1899, and this rose to over 350 just five years later. With the young age of the immigrants, and the relatively high birth rate, Glasgow Jewry was able to expand in the next decade or two by natural growth, as well as by the continuation of immigration, though this became less important in the years after the First World War. By the eve of the First World War there were about 12,000 Jews in Glasgow. The Jewish population was rising by about 300 each year with a greater proportion of the increase coming from natural growth. While there were still many Jewish newcomers arriving in the city in the first years of the twentieth century, there was also significant emigration as Jews moved on to England and especially to the United States of America.

The Jewish community was also becoming recognised as an integral part of the life of the city. Some of the credit for this may be attributed to the role of Michael Simons, who was certainly the best-known Glasgow Jew in the wider community and a role model for Jews who saw economic advance as an attainable aspiration. Although born in London in 1842, Simons had lived in Glasgow from the age of five years, and had contributed much to the life of the city. He was an eloquent spokesman for the Jewish community and had once been offered the position of Lord Provost, which he had declined. He had served on some important municipal committees and had taken charge of several of the committees involved in the organisation of the Glasgow Exhibitions of 1890 and 1901.[43]

Gorbals Jewry, too, learned the lesson of the value of close contacts with the city authorities. Soon there was municipal funding for the provision of English language teaching for the new immigrants, and from 1885 the Gorbals Bathhouse made provision of a *mikva,* a Jewish ritual bath, the first south of the river, and the only one in the Gorbals until the opening of the Great Synagogue in South Portland Street in 1901. A further recognition of the Jewish position in the city came in May 1902 when the City Chamberlain contacted Garnethill Synagogue, informing them that they wished 'to co-operate with the Jewish authorities' and were willing to provide 'a substantial dinner for deserving (poor Jewish) residents of the South Side'.[44] The City Chamberlain said that they wished to show that all sections of the city population should share in the life of Glasgow without regard to race or creed. Garnethill gratefully accepted the offer and set up a committee to choose those who would attend.

These years saw rapid growth in every area of community life. New synagogues appeared in the Gorbals. Jewish bakehouses and bakeries, fish and poultry shops and butchers, groceries and dairies provided a supply of kosher food. In addition, Jews were becoming a noticeable part of the Glasgow scene as unemployed immigrants congregated on Gorbals streets. As we shall see, a large number of Jewish welfare agencies catered for the requirements of the newcomers and tried to provide facilities that established them as productive members of their new community while meeting their religious and ethnic needs.

The Aliens Issue

However, the wider area of the general conditions of Jewish life can only be considered against the background of the immigration issue. This first surfaced in the 1890s as the numbers of Jewish aliens increased, especially in London's East End, Manchester and Leeds. Immigrant Jews had become a noticeable element in Britain's major cities. Their presence caused alarm to the established Jewish community, concerned that their own hard-won status would be affected by the newcomers, and that communal philanthropy might actually be increasing the level of immigration, by providing an attraction to destitute Jews. Those who wished to limit Jewish immigration included, by the 1890s, a small but influential Jewish lobby. The policy of the London Jewish Board of Guardians (LJBG) to repatriate poor and destitute Jews only made sense in the context of limiting the influx. In addition, the LJBG attempted to differentiate between 'genuine refugees', who might contribute to the wellbeing of the country, and 'undesirables with diseases and criminality'.[45]

In Glasgow, some minor repatriation was organised by the Board of Guardians but numbers were very small, said to be just a 'family or two or perhaps a few individuals' and certainly not on the scale of the 50,000 men, women and children returned by the LJBG to Eastern Europe between 1880 and 1914. In Glasgow, it was emphasised that repatriation was only done as last resort and with the full consent of those concerned.[46] The LJBG also protested they were committed only to voluntary repatriation, emphasising that even the return of half the Rumanian *fusgayers*, thousands of whom had marched in desperation from Rumania across Europe, in 1900 was 'mainly at their own request and naturally, never without their own consent'.[47]

The records of the Glasgow Hebrew Philanthropic Society show that aid for Jewish family reunion, whether in America, England or on the Continent, was provided from the 1870s especially when newcomers had shown an inability to provide for themselves and their families. In September 1881 a Jewish immigrant was given tickets for himself, his wife and son to Hamburg after '. . . he tried to travel with pictures, but after hawking about for a week he had earned nothing'.[48]

Health issues also played a part. In Glasgow immigrant health, and in particular the fear of the eye disease trachoma, was just one factor in the call for limitation of alien immigration. There was to be no consensus on the health of the immigrants. There were detractors like Harry Lawson, Conservative MP for Mile End in London, who referred to the immigration as a 'backward march to physical deterioration'.[49] On the other, and more supportive, side the Liberal MP Charles Rolleston considered that 'the Israelite is proving himself to be a regenerating force and a most useful acquisition to our citizenship'.[50]

One of the leading campaigners for a limit to the Jewish immigration was Major W.E. Evans-Gordon M.P. who took a consistently anti-alien line. Evans-Gordon wrote a book entitled *The Alien Immigrant* and actually visited Lithuania to assess the conditions of the Jewish population there in an attempt to influence the Royal Commission on Alien Immigration in 1903.[51] He could not see the point of transferring the wretched poor of the ghetto in Vilna to the slums of London's East End especially as some of the Jews he met had already been sent back to Vilna by the LJBG, as part of their repatriation policy.[52] Describing some of the conditions, he found that it reminded him

> . . . strongly, of a poor Scotch village. The people (of the suburbs of Slobodka) looked more healthy and robust than those of the ghettoes in the towns. The interior arrangements of the houses were similar to those of a Scotch croft. Some of the floors were without boards and plastered with mud.[53]

The Royal Commission provided an opportunity for both sides to present their views on the merits of the immigration. Jews were not the only immigrants, but as the first significant group of non-Christian immigrants to Britain some of their folk customs, religious practices and behaviour patterns must have seemed strange. Holmes has pointed out the evidence for anti-Semitism as part of the anti-alien hostility.[54] Jewish social separateness was adduced as proof, for example by eugenists, that Jews could never integrate into British life: '. . . for such men as religion, social habits or language keep as a caste apart there should be no place'.[55] Some expressed the feeling that 'all had been well' before the Jews had arrived, and many of those giving evidence to the Royal Commission, and especially those from the East End of London, showed varying degrees of anti-Jewish hostility.[56]

Julius Pinto and Jacob Kramrisch gave evidence to the Commission on behalf of the Glasgow Jewish community.[57] Pinto was concerned to show the size of the Jewish population in Scotland accurately and to comment fairly on their housing and economic situation, while giving an account of local Jewish achievements. Pinto pointed to the few prosecutions against Jews for overcrowded houses and said that he had been authorised by the Chief Sanitary Inspector to say that immigrant Jewish housing compared favourably with their neighbours as regards cleanliness. Pinto was speaking against a background of anti-alien propaganda in Glasgow as a pamphlet, entitled *Undesirable Aliens*, was being sold freely on the streets. This purported to deal with the alleged fraud of the Guitar Zither Company which had been been established in 1899 by a number of Rumanian Jews at the time of the *fusgayers*' march across Europe.[58]

Pinto showed how the wearing of ready-made suits had become more widely available in Scotland only as a result of the cost reductions obtained by Jewish methods of manufacture.[59] The changes had not been achieved, he considered, by sweated labour but by the better organisation of Jewish tailoring. In addition, the demand for skilled operatives continued to outstrip the supply, pushing up the piecework wages. While Jewish tailors developed pieceworking, the Scottish tailor still completed the entire garment himself, serving a different and more expensive market. Further, the credit method of selling helped to sustain the growth of the community, attracting more Jewish tailors to the city. Pinto accused the large firm of Stewart and MacDonald of being the real sweaters in Glasgow, despite their spacious factory, as their practice of contracting out work to Jewish tailors, at strictly controlled prices, was perpetuating the sweating system.

Kramrisch, Austrian-born Jewish manager, since 1888, of the Stephen Mitchell and Sons branch of the Imperial Tobacco Company, was closely involved with the development of Jewish activity in the cigarette industry.[60] While early recruitment of Jews into tobacco work had been slow, by the early years of the twentieth century it had become one of the major employers of Jewish labour in Glasgow. There were over 200 Jewish cigarette workers, some of whom were very highly skilled, and the concentration of cigarette manufacture in Glasgow had led to increased job opportunities in the ancillary packaging, printing and box-making areas. Kramrisch felt that the Glasgow tobacco trade was dependent on foreign labour and would not have come into being without it. In fact he had recruited Jewish workers directly from Russia and Germany, although latterly there had been a number of Jewish tobacco workers from Russia and Poland who had emigrated to London and Manchester and they had been brought from there to Glasgow by Kramrisch.

The United Synagogue of Glasgow acted as the local representative Jewish body in opposing the Aliens Bill and lobbied all the Glasgow MPs.[61] The only public test of Jewish opinion in Glasgow on the subject of alien immigration was the debate held by the Jewish Literary Society, based substantially on the Garnethill membership in February 1903.[62] Though Bertie Heilbronn represented those who felt that the limitation of immigration would safeguard the position of Jews already in Britain, it was the opposing view which carried overwhelming support.

Liberal opposition to the Aliens Bill during 1904 led to a considerable watering down, or even elimination, of its strictest provisions before it became law. When in power the Liberal Government refused to enforce its provisions strictly, so in the end the Act really only prevented the arrival of destitute travellers. Jewish immigration did fall after 1906 but not as significantly as many often suppose, though the placing of the Act on the statute book may have affected the attitudes of potential immigrants in

Eastern Europe.[63] Immigration control was confined to ships carrying more than twelve aliens docking at one of fourteen designated British ports, including Leith. Those who were ill, had insufficient funds, that is less than £5, or who did not possess transmigrant tickets, were to be refused admission. Yet there were significant numbers of Jews still coming to Glasgow who could meet the entry criteria.

The first person to fall foul of the new regulations was a traveller to Glasgow, Chana Gluckstein, coming from Russia to join her son.[64] She had contravened the new regulations on two counts. Firstly, she had only 6/- with her and was also suffering from the skin condition of lupus. Despite an appeal she was deported to Hamburg. Appeals against exclusion were not only possible but were often successful.[65] A couple were admitted to Britain, after a long wait pending appeal, despite the wife having trachoma, to join their daughter in a two-bedroom tenemental flat in Glasgow.[66] This had the permission of the Medical Officer of Health who stipulated that a separate room be provided for the newcomer. Thus, in the end the numbers excluded by the Aliens Act were so few that it was strange that there had been so much fuss.

References

1 James Cleland, *Enumeration of the Inhabitants of the City of Glasgow and the County of Lanark for the Government Census of 1831*, pp.72–73,188.
2 Charles W J Withers, *Urban Highlanders: Highland-Lowland Migration and Urban Gaelic Culture 1700–1900* (East Linton, 1998), p.4.
3 C C Aronsfeld, 'German Jews in Dundee', *Jewish Chronicle*, 20/11/1953.
4 *Records of Scottish Bankruptcies*, National Archives for Scotland, Edinburgh.
5 *Jewish Chronicle*, 25/4/1856: 25/7/1856: 16/10/1857.
6 *Glasgow Herald*, 7/9/1858.
7 James Brown, 'An Account of the Jews in Glasgow City 11/9/1858', in *The Religious Denominations of Glasgow*, Volume 1 (Glasgow, 1860), pp.4,11.
8 First Annual Report of the Committee of the Cemetery to the Merchants' *House*, Glasgow, 9/6/1835, Mitchell Library, Glasgow; David Daiches, *Glasgow* (London, 1977), p.139; A. Levy, *Origins of Glasgow Jewry 1812–1895* (Glasgow, 1949), pp.23–30.
9 *The Conversion of the Jews* (Edinburgh, 1842), pp.vi,51.
10 Kenneth E Collins, *Second City Jewry: the Jews of Glasgow in the age of Expansion 1790–1919* (Glasgow, 1990), pp.44, 72–73.
11 Minutes of the Glasgow Hebrew Congregation (GHC) 18/3/1866, Scottish Jewish Archives Centre, SJAC, Garnethill Synagogue, Glasgow.

12 Evidence of Julius Pinto to Royal Commission on Alien immigration (1903), 20854–20998: Letter (13/10/1875) to Michael Simon, Hon. Secretary, GHC, from Arthur and Company, Queen Street, Glasgow. Filed in GHC Letters Book, SJAC.
13 *Jewish Chronicle*, 12/11/1875: 19/11/1875.
14 *Jewish Chronicle*, 2/9/1881.
15 Kenneth Collins, *op.cit.*, p.36.
16 *Ibid.*, pp.42–43: 49–54.
17 Bill Williams, *The Making of Manchester Jewry 1740–1875* (Manchester, 1985), p.273.
18 *Jewish Chronicle*, 19/8/1881.
19 *Jewish Chronicle*, 2/9/1881.
20 Kenneth Collins, *op.cit.*, p.54.
21 *Ibid.*, p.49.
22 Kenneth Collins, 'United Synagogue of Glasgow 1898–1906', in *Second City Jewry, op.cit.*, pp.83–100.
23 *Ibid.*, pp.95–97.
24 *Jewish Chronicle*, 19/12/1913.
25 *Jewish Chronicle*, 19/8/1881.
26 Kenneth Collins, *op.cit.*, pp.64–66.
27 *Jewish Chronicle*, 3/2/1882.
28 Kenneth E. Collins, ed., *Aspects of Scottish Jewry* (Glasgow, 1987), pp.37–40.
29 Gorbals Public School Log 1890–1900, Strathclyde Archives, Mitchell Library, Glasgow.
30 Reports of the Glasgow Sanitary Department 1906–1914, Glasgow City Archives, Mitchell Library.
31 Kenneth Collins, *op.cit.*, p.38.
32 Lloyd P Gartner, *The Jewish Immigrant in England 1870–1914* (London, 1973), p.36–37.
33 *Jewish Chronicle*, 24/7/1891.
34 *Jewish Chronicle*, 16/10/1891.
35 *Jewish Chronicle*, 23/10/1891.
36 *Jewish Chronicle*, 14/8/1891.
37 *Jewish Chronicle*, 18/9/1891.
38 Kenneth Collins, *Second City Jewry,* p.66.
39 *Jewish Chronicle*, 16/10/1891.
40 Reports of the Glasgow Sanitary Department 1906–1914, Glasgow City Archives, Mitchell Library.
41 Minutes of the Garnethill Hebrew Congregation, 29/5/1910, SJAC.
42 Register of Births, Marriages and Deaths, Glasgow Hebrew Congregation, SJAC.
43 Charles Winston, *Lodge Montefiore No.753: 1888–1988* (Glasgow,1988), pp.3–5.
44 *Jewish Chronicle*, 23/5/1902.
45 Geoffrey Alderman, *Modern British Jewry* (Oxford, 1992), pp.134–5.
46 Kenneth Collins, *op.cit.*, p.71.
47 Chaim Bermant, *Troubled Eden: An Anatomy of British Jewry* (London, 1969), p.25.
48 Ben Braber, Integration of Jewish Immigrants in Glasgow 1880–1939, University of Glasgow unpublished PhD thesis (1992), p.30–31.

49 John A Garrard, *The English and Immigration 1880–1910* (London, 1971), p.18.
50 *Ibid.*, p.19.
51 Report of the Royal Commission on Alien Immigration (1903), evidence of Major W E Evans-Gordon, 26/2/1903.
52 Chaim Bermant, *Troubled Eden* (London, 1969), pp.25–27.
53 Report of the Royal Commission on Alien Immigration (1903), evidence of Major W E Evans-Gordon, 26/2/1903.
54 Colin Holmes, *Anti-Semitism in British Society 1876–1939* (London, 1979), p.18
55 Karl Pearson and Margaret Moul, 'The Problem of Alien Immigration into Great Britain, Illustrated by an Examination of Russian and Polish Jewish Children', *Annals of Eugenics*, 1925/5, p.125.
56 Colin Holmes, *op.cit.*,p.18.
57 Report of the Royal Commission on Alien Immigration (1903), evidence of Julius Pinto 20854–20998; evidence of Jacob Kramrisch 21714–21738.
58 *Jewish Chronicle*, 2/10/1903.
59 Report of the Royal Commission on Alien Immigration (1903), evidence of Julius Pinto, 20854–20874.
60 Report of the Royal Commission on Alien Immigration (1903), evidence of Jacob Kramrisch, 21714–21738.
61 Minutes of the United Synagogue 1898–1906, 21/6/1905, at SJAC.
62 *Jewish Chronicle*, 6/2/1903.
63 Geoffrey Alderman, *The Jewish Community in British Politics* (Oxford,1983), pp.77–78.
64 *Jewish Chronicle*, 22/6/1906.
65 Gerry Black, Health and Medical Care of the Jewish Poor in the East End of London: 1880–1939, unpublished PhD thesis, University of Leicester 1987, p.22.
66 *Jewish Chronicle*, 3/4/1908.

CHAPTER TWO

Social Aspects of Health

'It is generally supposed that Jews have never been able to get a good footing in Scotland. The Scotch, it is urged, are 'too cannie'. Undoubtedly, there is some force in this argument; but, nevertheless, Jews, and even Polish Jews have, of recent years, found their way north of the Tweed.'
The Lancet, 23rd June 1888, p.1261

Assimilation and Acculturation

There was much about the new immigrants that made them distinctive, and thus they posed a threat to the position of the existing community. Jews, however, were not the only distinctive newcomers in Glasgow. Withers has described the cultural differences of the Gaelic-speaking Highlander settling in the Scottish Lowlands. The migrant status is therefore seen as a dynamic and mediating mechanism, between the society being transformed, and an urbanising society, itself subject to great change.[1] As Williams has pointed out, assimilation could be restricted in a society where Jewish immigrants worked long hours together, returning from their cramped workshops to a close-knit residential area, while their children spent every free hour in a communal *cheder*.[2]

While Jews around Garnethill set great store by blending carefully into their environment, the Jews in the Gorbals created a district within Glasgow that reminded them of *der heim*. Chaim Bermant described it thus many years later:

> There were Yiddish posters on the hoardings, Hebrew lettering on the shops, Jewish names, Jewish faces, Jewish butchers, Jewish bakers with Jewish bread, and Jewish grocers with barrels of herring in the doorway. One heard Yiddish in the streets . . . and one encountered figures who would not have been out of place in Barovke.[3]

Lewis Grassic Gibbon and Hugh Macdiarmid visited the Gorbals and described its Jewish aspects:

> . . . it is not even a Scottish slum. Stout men in beards and ringlets and unseemly attire lounge and strut with pointed shoes: Ruth and Naomi go by with downcast eastern faces . . . it is haunted by an ancient ghost of goodness and grossness, sunwarmed and ripened under alien suns.[4]

While this Yiddish milieu persisted in the Gorbals, there was pressure, even prejudice, against the pervasive use of the Yiddish language by the new immigrants. Yiddish was often referred to in a derogatory fashion as 'jargon' or *Judisch-deutsch*. While the Gaelic Highlander could maintain his tongue as the language of prayer in his urban chapels, the Jewish immigrant used Hebrew, rather than Yiddish, at prayer. Rev. Simeon Singer, compiler of the standard Jewish Daily Prayer Book, speaking at the opening of a new Gorbals synagogue in September 1892, hoped that Gorbals Jewry would not use Yiddish 'an hour longer than you can help', calling it 'a mixture of bad German and bad Hebrew'.[5] Children were often embarrassed by the foreignness of their parents. Rev. Levine, the assistant minister at Garnethill, described the 'weaknesses' of the immigrant Jews as 'due to the environment of their earlier days in countries such as Russia', claiming that some of their customs were actually counter to the laws of the *Shulchan Aruch*, the Jewish religious code.[6]

In the Gorbals a wide variety of Jewish after-school education was available, mostly taught in the Yiddish language. The main religion classes were provided by the Talmud Torah, founded in Clyde Street in 1895 and supported both by Garnethill Synagogue and Gorbals Jewry.[7] Enrolment at the Talmud Torah reached 376 pupils in 1908 when the Great Synagogue in South Portland Street decided to open its own religion classes with English as the language of instruction.[8] The move was controversial and opposed by some of the more traditionalist teachers. The Gaels had found that preservation of urban Gaelic depended more on the existence of Gaelic-speaking churches than on direct transmission down the generations.[9] With the pressure to learn English to succeed at school and in employment, Jewish families were speaking less Yiddish at home. Children only spoke Yiddish at home if their parents could not speak adequate English, and the religion classes remained as the one means of passing on the Yiddish language to the next generation. When the religion classes switched to the medium of the English language, the days of Yiddish were numbered.

One potential bulwark against assimilation might have been the provision of a Jewish school in the Gorbals.[10] At a time when the Jewish pupils made up a high proportion of the children in Gorbals schools, schemes were proposed to make one of the city schools a Jewish school. Such efforts foundered primarily because of opposition within the school authorities. An attempt was made before the First World War to set up a Hebrew language school in the Gorbals. Beginning as evening classes, it had neither the premises nor support to become a permanent institution. Despite these factors the Yiddish language did survive for a long time. As late as 1919 a Glasgow Jewish Library Council was established to provide Yiddish material for those Jews, still estimated to be a majority of the community, who were only literate in Hebrew and Yiddish.[11] Yet, in one generation Glasgow Jewry's acculturation in dress, language, culture, social habits and, for many, their Russian-sounding surnames, was complete.

Given the social conditions in much of the Gorbals, there is remarkably little evidence of communal antagonism. Ralph Glasser, in describing his memories of an 'oppressive' anti-Semitism based on immigrant memories of attitudes encountered in the countries of origin, wrote that in Glasgow it was 'far from as violent and as publicly condoned'.[12] Consequently, when episodes of violence did occur, they received wide attention. In September 1912, ten boys were arrested and their fathers each fined a guinea after a fight between Jewish and gentile boys in Adelphi Street.[13] There had been some damage to property, mostly broken windows, but there was no physical injury. Baillie MacMillan who judged the case commented on 'parents allowing their children to run wild'. In an interview with the *Jewish Chronicle* in March 1911 Michael Simons commented on the level of anti-Jewish prejudice in Glasgow. Simons felt that the initial problems with housing and overcrowding had been settled within the previous few years.[14] The depressed housing market and the shortage of suitable accommodation in the Gorbals had led to some friction although Pinto's evidence to the Royal Commission on Alien Immigration in 1903 and Michael Simons' interview in 1911 both discounted substantial overcrowding.[15]

Clearly what made Jews distinctive was their religion. Although the level of adherence to traditional Jewish practices tended to decline with time, the mass of the community remained overwhelmingly loyal in its affiliation to Orthodox Judaism. The moderate form of Jewish Orthodoxy, at Garnethill, was respected by the newcomers. It was used as their model when Jews moved southwards out of the Gorbals to areas like Queens Park and preserved Orthodoxy as the predominant Jewish religious stream in Glasgow. While Gorbals Jewry campaigned for many years before the First World War for a 'foreign born *Rav*' to lead their community in a more traditionalist manner, this was not at the expense of the Rev. E.P. Phillips, minister at Garnethill from 1879, who had been recognised as the religious leader for all Glasgow Jewry by the Chief Rabbi before Glasgow Jewry's major growth had occurred.

Sabbath observance and adherence to a kosher diet outside the home were often the first practices under pressure from the society round about, and even in the early days intermarriage, while limited, was still a feature.[16] Jewish after-school education and Jewish youth activities were a priority for a community unable to establish a Jewish day school. Even at Garnethill, where there had been considerable experimentation with the synagogue service, including the use of a mixed voice choir, there was no doubt about their lasting attachment to Orthodoxy.[17] Indeed, it was not until the 1930s, and the beginnings of immigration from Germany, that a small Reform congregation was established in Glasgow. However, Glasgow Jewry on the whole steered a balance between maintaining the traditional patterns of Jewish life while substantially integrating into Glaswegian society.

Employment

Any complacency about social and working conditions of the new Jewish community in Glasgow was dispelled by an investigation conducted in the autumn of 1888 by a Special Sanitary Commission reporting in the medical journal, *The Lancet*.[18] This investigation, covering many of the major cities in Britain, provided a savage indictment of the conditions in the sweated workshops, many of them Jewish-owned, which had sprung up since about 1875. In Glasgow, Scots and Irish migrants were involved, as well as Jews, in the sweating trades. These exploited younger workers and tied them into a form of labour from which there was little escape.

Sweating usually meant long hours of work with poor pay in unhealthy workshops. The work done by sweated workers was usually partly-made goods to be finished in premises outside the factory. One of the evils consequent on sweating was subcontracting which isolated and marginalised workers, but it could provide quick access for poorly skilled newcomers, such as Jewish immigrants, to the labour market. Further, it could provide the opportunity for sweated workers to progress beyond their current daily grind into a more prosperous future. But for the inexperienced young workers, by the time they were conversant with the methods of labour they would be dismissed so that the next batch of newcomers could be 'trained' for employment.[19]

The Lancet report may have suffered from some exaggeration but there had to be some answers for a system that promoted such widespread abuse:

> To be overcrowded, poor, half-starved in ill-ventilated, insufficiently lighted, over-crowded, over-heated, and badly drained workshops is evil enough; but to be compelled to work in the same courts, to pass under the same narrow, dark, low passages where half-drunken women stand listlessly about, to be surrounded by vice, which in Glasgow has

> reached the last expression of degradation and bestiality, is a danger, a humiliation, an insult against honest workers and against womankind at large, which should evoke the indignation and shame of the entire community.

The Commission noted the effects on poor Jewish immigrants and their families. These immigrants were trying to set up small businesses for themselves, often working from their own inadequate apartments. They were often caught up in overcrowded and insanitary conditions, and the only solution for the authorities seemed to be the application of health and hygiene standards. Not unexpectedly, the *Lancet* report on sweated labour in Glasgow, published just a week after its assessment of the situation in Edinburgh, caused considerable anxiety in Glasgow. With its use of lurid language, exaggeration of Jewish numbers and racial stereotyping, there seemed much to fear:

> The Jews of Glasgow are now thoroughly on the alert, and seem to feel that their position is seriously menaced. For the first time during these investigations we were flatly refused admittance into one sweated workshop.[20]

Though a public meeting was held in Glasgow in October 1888 to air the problems described in the *Lancet* and to allow 'public indignation to be expressed', the issue did not attract overwhelming public attention. The hall was far from full and no mention was made of any ethnic aspect of the system, given the then small size of the Jewish community and the presence, identified in the *Lancet*, of 'exceptionally large numbers' of Scots and Irish, rather than Jews, in Glasgow's sweated workshops.[21]

Julius Pinto, in giving evidence to the Select Committee set up by the House of Lords following the *Lancet* report, claimed that agitation against the Jewish tailors was nothing more than an 'outcry' by local tailors for some protection of their interests.[22] Indeed, we have already seen that he accused one major local clothing firm, operating from a large factory, of encouraging sweating by subcontracting to Jewish workshops. He noted that there had been only two convictions against Jewish tailors under the Factory Act and none under the Public Health Act. Pinto was supported by George Sedgewick, HM Factory Inspector, who had found conditions in Jewish factories and workshops to be 'fair', and not lacking in cleanliness as Dr. James Russell, Glasgow Medical Officer of Health, had alleged, though less so when home and workplace were combined. Pinto blamed some of the agitation on reactions to Jewish tailoring innovations, while his view of the Scottish working man was quite unflattering:

> . . . the native working man has nothing to fear from his foreign competitors if only he would adapt himself to improvements of the trade, and not adhere to his antiquated method of production. If he would discontinue his worship of Bacchus and his celebration of St. Mondays and St. Tuesdays, and if he would study the interests of his employers more than he does that of football and the sporting papers he would have nothing at all to dread from the foreign competitor.[23]

Scottish trade unions remained supportive of the immigrant workers, understanding the pressures facing Jewish tailors and their working practices. There is, for example, the following statement made about a Jewish tailoring firm which relocated to Glasgow in 1893, taking many jobs with them: 'If they were hunted out of their own country the chief duty of trade unions was to get them into the trade unions and have them working under the same conditions as their fellow-workers'.[24]

Writing just a few years later, in 1899, Mary Hancock reported her own investigations into alien trades, speaking at a meeting of the West of Scotland Branch of the Women's Liberal Association. She found that Jewish clothing workers had met new needs and that sweating allegations had been much exaggerated. In shoemaking she found that local shoemakers were not afraid of Jewish competitors who were making cheaper goods for a different clientele.[25]

The 1891 Census showed that Gorbals Jewry was still concentrated in a very few occupations, although in the ten years since the 1881 Census some real changes had occurred.[26] More Jews were working in other manufacturing activities outside tailoring and a significant group of shopkeepers had emerged. A large number were engaged in peddling, travelling to the mining villages of Ayrshire and Lanarkshire. This was an easy way of getting into business, and many successful shopkeepers began this way, often with start-up loans from one of the Jewish free loan societies. Pedlars were especially involved in the sale of cheap jewellery, clothing, lace and such household decorations as picture frames, obtained on easy credit terms from Glasgow warehouses, often without deposit. Peddling was still a major source of Jewish employment in Glasgow and Edinburgh well into the twentieth century, even after it had ceased to be a common Jewish occupation in London and Manchester.[27] Peddling inevitably declined as the Scottish retail system improved, and those still involved as pedlars became a more forlorn and impoverished group, economic failures that were unable to make the transition into retailing as the more successful had done.[28]

Some shop work was related to the provision and sale of kosher products but many more were drapers, jewellers or described themselves as general dealers. Only a small number became labourers or other unskilled workers, with a few finding employment in areas such as port work. Another group were blacksmiths who had followed that trade in Poland. Conditions were not easy: the pay, at £1.50 weekly, was better than might be obtained in Poland but the long eighty-hour week in the smithy would have sapped the energies of all but the strongest.[29] A small number of the women, usually unmarried relatives of other householders, worked as domestics but Census returns show that even in cramped Gorbals apartments many Jewish families had Scottish or Irish domestic servants. They might be expected to help in the small workshops, or were used to assist with the younger children to free the Jewish women and older children to do tailoring work.

The Jewish employment trends during the pre-War years continued in the pattern established in the previous two decades. A study of alien Jews working in factories and workshops in

Glasgow was conducted during 1908 by Miss Meiklejohn, an Inspector attached to the Glasgow Sanitary Department, who visited Jewish homes as well as over a hundred places where Jews were employed. She confirmed that Jews were mostly employed in just a few occupations. Tailoring was the only trade in which large numbers of Jewish women were employed and was the major employer of Jewish labour in Glasgow. About 500 Jewish men and women were working mainly in small workshops but there was some evidence of work sharing between different workshops.

Shoemaking was carried out in a network of small cobblers' shops in the Gorbals, which employed virtually only male workers. The high level of Jewish employment in cigarette making had dropped from its peak a few years earlier with the introduction of machinery into the factories. The number of Glasgow tobacco factories had not altered and the drop in employment affected native workers as well as the immigrant Jews. However, a considerable number of Jewish women were still said to be found in retail tobacconists selling and making cigarettes. Some married women kept shops while their husbands were employed in workshops or factories. There was little evidence of the Jewish women in the same work patterns as their gentile neighbours, and there was no evidence at all of home employment of children on any regular basis. For the first time cabinet making ranked as an important employer of Jewish labour with 200 men employed in two factories and eleven workshops. The sixty women employed in these Jewish-owned cabinet making businesses, mainly involved in French polishing, were all gentile because, it was said, Jewish women 'did not like the hard manual work entailed'.[30]

The Meiklejohn survey identified a problem with deserted wives. This problem was often related to the so-called secret marriages and divorces, known in Yiddish as *stille chuppas v'gittin.*[31] These marriages were conducted in many of the immigrant areas by rabbis who were immigrants themselves and who did not have official communal status. As they were arranged without reporting details to the civil registration bodies, they would have seemed attractive to newcomers unfamiliar with such requirements. Indeed, in the immigrant areas such unfamiliarity with registration procedures often led to delay in birth notification. In Glasgow, the United Synagogue had rebuked Rabbi Abraham Shyne, resident in the Gorbals for about twenty years, but without a synagogue pulpit, or recognised communal authority for conducting 'irregular divorces'.[32] Divorces, or marriages, which were conducted by Shyne were not recorded by the synagogue and would not have been supplied to the civil authorities. Thus there was no binding civil marriage or divorce contract and no protection for abandoned wives. Some of these abandoned wives had husbands in America and occasionally they received money sent back to support them and their families. In other cases women relied on the charity of the Board of Guardians or the Hebrew Ladies' Benevolent Society, which had to suffice until the children were able to support themselves and their mother. Little evidence of Jewish destitution was found and this was attributed to the efficient operation of 'the Jewish system of charity'.

Housing

One potential area of friction between the Jews and their neighbours was Jewish housing conditions in the Gorbals, the only district in Glasgow where Jewish residents formed a significant section of the local population. The poor Jewish reputation in housing was reflected in a survey of properties in the Gorbals Cross area in 1901, bequeathed to the University of Glasgow. The survey reported that 'unfortunately the properties are largely occupied by Jews who make very bad tenants, especially in neglecting needed repairs'.[33]

There were a number of studies of immigrant Jewry in the Gorbals that looked at issues such as housing, as well as immigration, employment and health. The Jewish community felt that it was important that information disseminated about Jews be based on proper investigation of the facts and not on emotional, superficial and inaccurate impressions. The community were naturally upset by prejudiced reports that exaggerated their numbers and gave false information about Jewish housing and health matters.

There were concerns that frankly anti-Semitic attitudes were especially noticeable in the rented housing market.[34] Jewish tenants encountered difficulties over the refusal of some factors to let houses to Jews in certain parts of the city, even though the loss on unlet property was small compared to what would be sustained by the owners of the property. Sometimes the other tenants in the tenement close expressed an aversion to the admission of a Jewish family, though many of the accusations made against Jews had no basis in fact.[35]

Housing problems continued to cause difficulties over many decades as Jews left the Gorbals seeking more salubrious accommodation in districts to the south as well as in the West End. The chosen method of dealing with this problem, a typical approach to many differing problems over the years, namely ‘a maximum of reasonable persistency and a minimum of fuss’, was slow in achieving results.[36] Some confirmation of the housing discrimination experienced by Jews in the Gorbals was detailed in a report of the Glasgow Municipal Commission on Housing for the Poor. One of those giving evidence was M. Gilmour, the Vice-President of the Association of House Factors and Property Agents, which had often put difficulties in the way of Jews seeking to let property. Gilmour alleged that the Jews who had settled in large numbers on the South Side of Glasgow had very insanitary habits.[37] He pointed to the increasing numbers of alien Jews in the Gorbals where farmed-out houses encouraged the migration of aliens and claimed that stairs and landings were not being properly cleaned.[38] Another agent giving evidence, P. Macaulay, told the Commission that he did not care to let property to Russian and Polish Jews.[39]

In fact, housing conditions had been notorious in the Glasgow slums long before the wave of Jewish immigration. There had been cholera outbreaks in the Glasgow slums in 1848/9 and 1853/4 causing many thousands of deaths. These epidemics were the spur to various housing improvements and demolition of the worst of the slums.[40] In addition, the opening of the Loch Katrine reservoir by Queen Victoria in 1859 guaranteed the city good clean water. However, with the Gorbals the home to so many thousands of newcomers there was continuing pressure on accommodation. Indeed, in an attempt to sweep the homeless off the streets a number of so-called 'model' lodging houses were built between 1871 and 1884 with one at Portugal Street in the Gorbals accommodating 437 of the city's most destitute inhabitants 'of all nationalities'.[41]

A system of 'ticketing' houses was introduced in 1886 for apartments of three rooms or less to try to prevent overcrowding. This legally limited the number of occupants allowed to live in these smaller homes. About one seventh of Gorbals houses were ticketed but there was still evidence of overcrowding with large families occupying homes too small for them.[42] In some, the overcrowding was attributed solely to lodgers but in a further third there was a combination of large families and lodgers. It was not always possible for inspectors to verify overcrowding, and in any case overcrowding could also be found in the larger apartments where official restrictions did not apply. Ticketing was backed up by a system of inspection by Sanitary Inspectors who could call at any time and close overcrowded flats. The Gorbals area had a substantial number of smaller apartments, with one or two rooms, and with four families on each floor sharing one lavatory, many of these apartments showed signs of squalor with backcourts becoming areas of rotting refuse and mud. However, the Gorbals also had some more salubrious areas. Abbotsford Place, for example, on the southern fringe with its amply proportioned apartments remained a more middle-class haven until well after the First World War.

Peter Fyfe, the Sanitary Chief of the City of Glasgow, produced a number of reports on housing conditions in Glasgow. Writing in 1901, Fyfe found that Jews were under-represented in the worst of the regular Gorbals housing though relatively few were living in the best of the Gorbals housing stock on its southern fringes.[43] Fyfe's studies of one- and two-apartment tenement flats showed that on average 3.2 people shared a room in one-room flats while the two-room flats had on average 4.2 people. Attempts at stricter control of overcrowding in these smaller 'ticketed' homes were made in the 1890s.

The 1881 Census showed a higher percentage of Jews living in four-room flats than in 1891. It would appear from the later Census that those who had achieved a degree of prosperity were moving out of the area, as Julius Pinto had done, or had left Glasgow with some capital to finance ventures elsewhere. The large majority of the Gorbals tenement homes were of two or three rooms with only small numbers having four rooms or indeed living in a single-room apartment. The Census figures of 1891 showed that the concentration of people in the Gorbals Jewish homes was on the high side with 3.5 inhabitants on average in one-room apartments and on average 5.2 in two-room apartments.[44] However, even these figures were still lower than general figures for occupancy in the area some ten years later. Fyfe also showed that only a very few Jews lived in the dark and insanitary homes, known as the backlands, which were built in the backcourts of the regular tenement blocks. Light often did not penetrate into these, much cheaper, apartments whose front windows faced the rear of the regular tenements.[45]

A few illustrations of the different households obtained from the 1891 Census Returns will show some of the patterns of migration and settlement.[46] Solomon Hervitch, an employed slipper-maker born in Russia, came to Glasgow with his wife Sarah in about 1888 when their daughter Bella was born. Their oldest daughters Mary and Betsy had been born in Russia but their son Joseph was born in London in 1887. Their youngest daughter Leah, aged four months, had also been born in London, perhaps implying a brief return there in search of work or merely returning to family or friends to facilitate the birth. Solomon and Sarah and their five children occupied one room at 116 Thistle Street.

More comfortable surroundings were enjoyed by the Jacobs family at 99 South Portland Street. Hyman Jacobs had been involved in trying to prolong the use of the Glassford Street hall for regular services, and his opposition to the mixed-voice choir at Garnethill led him to become more active in the nascent Gorbals synagogue.[47] Jacobs had come to England with his wife Fanny and three young sons in about 1872 and their daughter Rachel had been born there. They left England for Glasgow in about 1875, where

Hyman and his older children all worked as tailors. Three more children were born in Glasgow, the first, Michael, in 1875, making a total of two adults and seven children living in a six-roomed apartment. A few doors along from the Jacobs, ironically, in the building later demolished to make way for the building of the South Portland Street Synagogue was Mauritz Michaelis, then 41 years old, the German-born self-styled 'Missionary to the Jews'.

Recent arrivals in Glasgow tended to settle in the one- or two-room apartments, often with a boarder or two to help with the rental costs. The minister of the Main Street Synagogue, Rev. Isaac Bridge, lived with his wife Fanny and four children, the younger two born in Glasgow, with a domestic servant in three rooms at 31 Norfolk Street. At 16 Main Street lived Barnet Lipschitz, the baker, with his wife and family. Lipschitz had reached Glasgow with his wife and oldest son Harris in about 1881 and by 1891 their family had increased to seven children. Sharing the three-room apartment were Sarah Myerovitch, an eighteen-year-old domestic from Russia, as well as a Scottish servant girl.

In his submission to the Royal Commission on Alien Immigration in 1903, Julius Pinto stated categorically that there was no overcrowding among the foreign Jews in Glasgow. He backed up his arguments by pointing both to the very few prosecutions by the Sanitary Department for overcrowding, including only one such prosecution in the previous two years, and referred to the Jewish immunity to serious diseases like smallpox and bubonic plague which had occurred in Thistle Street and Rose Street in the Gorbals in 1899, despite the large numbers of Jews residing in these streets.[48] Although the level of prosecutions under the ticketing regulations could not be an accurate reflection of housing conditions and the Census records confirm the level of occupancy of Jewish homes, Pinto insisted, on the basis of his own detailed investigations, that the Gorbals Jews, who lived mainly in small apartments, were not overcrowded. He stated that he was

> . . . authorised by the chief sanitary inspector to say that the houses of the foreign Jews compare favourably, as regards

> cleanliness, with those of the class among whom they reside, and it is pointed out by one of the inspectors that he invariably found their bed clothing much cleaner than that of their surrounding neighbours.[49]

Ralph Glasser's portrayal of incest in the Gorbals during the interwar years, described in his book *Growing up in the Gorbals*, aroused much controversy when it was published.[50] While it was felt that the closely knit Jewish family and community network militated against the social problems evident in the wider society, it would seem unlikely that all the Jewish families would be able to insulate themselves from their surroundings. Jews were living in areas where there were significant numbers of overcrowded homes where night-time accommodation had to be shared.

The scandal of Glasgow slum properties, some of them in the very areas where the immigrants were settling, was an issue for the Glasgow City Council and for the City Improvement Trust.[51] Dr. James Russell, Glasgow's Medical Officer of Health, who recognised the link between health and insanitary housing, some of which was clearly beyond repair, had spurred them into action in the mid-1880s. From 1896 Glasgow Corporation began to acquire land for housing and the Improvement Trust began the task of slum clearance and redevelopment. The worst of the housing would disappear but the twin pressures of poverty and overcrowding would continue to ensure that many of the Gorbals properties remained the worst of the city's housing stock.

Crime

There was a general consensus on the low level of crime and drunkenness within the Glasgow Jewish community. The Jewish population had a reputation with the police of being law-abiding, their main fault being a 'predisposition to quarrelsomeness among themselves'.[52] However, this did not mean a total absence of crime. While there were virtually no crimes of violence, criminality usually involved commercial dishonesty, like forgery and fraudulent bankruptcy.[53] In Edinburgh, for example, Rev. Furst conducted services on both days of Rosh Hashanah, the New Year, in the Calton Jail in September 1900 although the number of Jewish prisoners was not specified.[54] In the first years of the twentieth century Duke Street Prison in Glasgow had only had eighteen Jewish prisoners of whom thirteen received sentences for a variety of petty crimes.[55] Sentences ranged from six days up to the two prisoners who were sentenced to six months' imprisonment. Barlinnie received a similar number of Jewish prisoners but there were no Jews in the women's prison.

With large sections of Jewry on the move there were abandoned wives and daughters in many transmigrant centres left penniless and at the mercy of ruthless operators who sold them into prostitution in South America and Shanghai. Concern had been expressed during the early years of the twentieth century about the 'white slave trade' and in particular about the Jewish role in it.[56] At first there did not seem to be a high level of interest in the problem within Glasgow Jewry but, taking the lead from Claude Montefiore, a small group met privately in Glasgow and decided that the Glasgow Jewish community would have to take some action. The natural instinct, with this issue as with many others, was to keep a low profile and to avoid the possibility of any criticism of Glasgow Jewry. Montefiore felt that anti-Semitism would not result from the publicity resulting from openly combating the menace but was more likely to follow if the problem was known about but not confronted.[57] It was generally felt that the approach of working through the local non-denominational Scottish National Vigilance Association was the most appropriate but there was no progress on forming a local branch for some time.[58]

When the Scottish National Vigilance Association eventually met in Glasgow in March 1913, presided over by the Episcopal Bishop of Glasgow, it was agreed to form a Glasgow Jewish Committee under the auspices of the Association's general committee. It was also agreed that a special worker should be employed for the Jewish branch in Glasgow with the local Jewish community to subscribe £50 annually towards the costs of the worker, the remainder of the expenses being met by the Association.[59]

Diet

A major study of working-class diets was carried out in Glasgow in 1911 and 1912, on the pattern of a similar investigation in Edinburgh some years earlier.[60] The report on the eating habits of sixty Glasgow families, including five Jewish families, was conducted by Dorothy Lindsay, Carnegie Research Fellow at the University of Glasgow, under the auspices of the Corporation of the City of Glasgow. The families had their diet and food expenditure studied for a complete week. The rigour of the study may have affected the sample as many families may not have welcomed the detailed scrutiny that was entailed. In addition, the report indicates that many of the families, especially where there was a history of alcoholism, were on their best behaviour and attempted to show their domestic arrangements in the best light. It is unclear whether the five Jewish families studied, described as 'on the whole better off than most of the British families visited', were typical of Gorbals Jewry as a whole, given that most of the immigrants' homes were humbly, or shabbily, fitted out, short of beds, with few objects of beauty, and in use by day and night as workrooms.[61]

Lindsay described the style of living in the Jewish homes, which as noted below seems quite impressive, as being similar to that of the other homes studied, if a little larger on average. The women too were 'more grandly dressed'. In common with their neighbours, the kitchens were used as living-rooms while '. . . the parlours are wonderful rooms, with full suites of furniture, photographs, crystal or china ornaments, anti-macassars etc . . .' Four out of the five families studied had between seven and twelve members in the household and a family income of between £1.75 and £2 weekly. This put the Jewish families above the average of the whole group of sixty households surveyed, and 'the women boasted of the fact that they had a regular dinner each day'. Nevertheless, there were significant health problems within the Jewish group. One of the mothers had been ill. Many of the children were described as 'delicate' and one child with rickets was attending a special invalid school. As the Jewish families studied were all foreign-born and living in the Gorbals, it is likely that, even if they were not typical of Gorbals Jewry as a whole, they represented a considerable strand within it.

While there are no other contemporary Glasgow studies including Jews, a few years earlier a study had been carried out of over a thousand Edinburgh schoolchildren in the poorest areas of the city, with children from two Jewish families.[62] One of the families (no.115) had managed to extricate themselves from dire poverty by 'keeping a rag shop and making slippers'. The family were well fed and were described as 'quiet and sober and liked by their neighbours'. The other family (no.488) were reported as being 'grimy, overcrowded and ill smelling', and the father had had a conviction for arson and was now a hawker. No health problems were reported in either home.

The Jewish families examined in the survey consumed three times as much fish as their non-Jewish neighbours yet spent more money on meat, partly attributed to the higher costs of kosher meat. There was also great reliance on chicken and Lindsay displayed great admiration for the family of ten who made half a chicken the high point of their Friday evening meal. With no problems of alcohol excess the Jewish families managed their diets well and the Jewish women appeared to have a better grasp of economics than the other Gorbals women. Hardy notes that the immigrant Jews in London too made use of a wide variety of healthy foodstuffs, not sharing the 'British preoccupation' with meat.[63] The main criticism of the Jewish diet was that the energy value for money expended was small compared with the diet of the Scottish families.

The conclusion of the study, that the poor should abandon meat, fish and eggs as too expensive and concentrate on a diet of porridge and milk, supplemented by cheese and cheap protein-rich vegetables, seems unduly patronising.[64] So too was the suggestion that instruction be given on the use of porridge and vegetables in schools along with the circulation of such booklets as *How to Spend a Shilling on Food to the Best Advantage* and *How to Feed a Family of Five on 12/9 a Week*. The Jewish families emerged from the study showing that they understood the key principles of a balanced diet and that despite health problems their food intake was on the whole satisfactory.

References

1 Charles W J Withers, *Urban Highlanders: Highland-Lowland Migration and Urban Gaelic Culture, 1700–1900* (East Linton, 1998), p.12.
2 Bill Williams, *The Making of Manchester Jewry 1740–1875* (Manchester, 1985), p.271.
3 Chaim Bermant, *Coming Home* (London, 1976), pp.52–53.
4 L Grassic Gibbon and Hugh Macdiarmid, 'Glasgow', in *Scottish Scene* (Glasgow, 1934).
5 *Jewish Chronicle*, 16/9/1892.
6 *Jewish Chronicle*, 9/4/1913.
7 Kenneth Collins, *Second City Jewry: the Jews of Glasgow in the Age of Expansion 1790–1919* (Glasgow, 1990), pp.75–77.
8 *Jewish Chronicle*, 4/6/1909.
9 Charles W J Withers, *op.cit.*, p.241.
10 Kenneth Collins, *op.cit.*, pp.131–133.
11 *Jewish Chronicle*, 6/6/1919.
12 Ralph Glasser, *Gorbals Boy at Oxford* (London, 1988), p.25.
13 *Jewish Chronicle*, 27/9/1912.
14 'Glasgow's Foremost Jew: an Interview with Michael Simons', in *Jewish Chronicle*, 24/3/1911.
15 *Ibid*; Report of the Royal Commission on Alien Immigration (1903), evidence of Julius Pinto, 20854–20874.
16 *Jewish Chronicle*, 8/11/1918.
17 *Jewish Chronicle*, 29/5/1914 and 24/12/1909.
18 'Report of the Lancet Special Sanitary Commission on the Sweating System in Edinburgh', *Lancet*, 23/8/1888, pp.1261–1262; 'Report of the Lancet Special Sanitary Commission on the Sweating System in Glasgow', *Lancet*, 30/6/1888, pp.1313–1314.
19 James A Schmiechen, *Sweated Industries and Sweated Labor: The London Clothing Trades 1860–1914* (London, 1984), pp.1–5.
20 'Report of the Lancet Special Sanitary Commission on the Sweating System in Glasgow', *op.cit.*, p.1313.
21 *Glasgow Herald*, 10/10/1888.
22 Sessional Papers of the House of Lords, Session 1889, Vol.VIII, evidence of Julius Pinto, 26206; George Sedgewick, 26455; Dr. James Russell, 26363.
23 Report of the Royal Commission on Alien Immigration, 1903, evidence of Julius Pinto, 20919.
24 Angela Tuckett, *The Scottish Trades Union Congress: the First 80 Years* (Edinburgh,1986), p.47.
25 *Jewish Chronicle*, 17/2/1899.
26 Census of Scotland for 1891, Gorbals District, Register House, Edinburgh.
27 Lloyd P Gartner, *The Jewish Immigrant in England 1870–1914* (London, 1973), p.60.
28 David Daiches, *Two Worlds* (Sussex, 1971), p.117.
29 Interview, Maurice Tobias, 1988, quoted in Kenneth Collins, *Second City Jewry: the Jews of Glasgow in the Age of Expansion* (Glasgow, 1990), p.63.
30 *Jewish Chronicle*, 31/7/1908.
31 Rainer Liedtke, *Jewish Welfare in Hamburg and Manchester c1850–1914*

(Oxford 1998), pp.155–156.
32 Rabbi Shyne did not receive a salary for his rabbinic activities and subsisted on collections of small sums made for him in the Gorbals. In an attempt to reduce his dependence on marriage and divorce fees an annual subvention of £25 a year was made to him from 1904. See Kenneth Collins, *op.cit.*, pp.88–89, 138; Minutes of the United Synagogue, 25/6/1900, 23/10/1904.
33 Kenneth Collins, *op.cit.*, p.164.
34 *Ibid.*
35 *Jewish Chronicle*, 22/7/1910.
36 'Glasgow's Most Prominent Jew: Interview with Michael Simons', *Jewish Chronicle,* 24/3/1911.
37 *Glasgow Municipal Commission on Housing for the Poor* (Glasgow, 1904), in Glasgow City Archives, Mitchell Library, pp.352,358.
38 *Ibid.*, p.255.
39 *Ibid.*, p.547.
40 Frank Worsdall, *The Tenement, A Way of Life: A Social, Historical and Architectural Study of Housing in Glasgow* (Edinburgh, 1979), p.7.
41 *Ibid.*, p.8.
42 *Annual Report of the Sanitary Department* (Glasgow, 1898), in Glasgow City Archives, Mitchell Library.
43 Peter Fyfe, *Backlands and their Inhabitants* (Glasgow, 1901), p.15.
44 Kenneth Collins, *op.cit.,* pp.222–224.
45 Report of the Royal Commission on Alien Immigration (1903), evidence of Julius Pinto, 20991–20998.
46 Census of Scotland for 1891, Gorbals District, Register House, Edinburgh.
47 Kenneth Collins, *op.cit.,* p.64.
48 Kenneth Collins, *op.cit.*, p.108.
49 Report of the Royal Commission on Alien Immigration (1903), evidence of Julius Pinto, 20871–20874.
50 Ralph Glasser, *Growing up in the Gorbals* (London,1986), pp.132–133.
51 Edna Robertson, *Glasgow's Doctor, James Burn Russell 1837–1904* (East Linton,1998), pp.160–162.
52 Royal Commission, *op.cit.*, evidence of Julius Pinto, 20895.
53 Lloyd P Gartner, *op.cit.*, p.183; Kenneth Collins, *op.cit.*, p.112.
54 *Jewish Chronicle*, 8/9/1900.
55 Royal Commission, *op.cit.*, evidence of Julius Pinto, 20895.
56 *Jewish Chronicle*, 2/4/1910.
57 *Jewish Chronicle*, 7/10/1910.
58 *Jewish Chronicle*, 3/1/1913.
59 *Jewish Chronicle*, 7/3/1913.
60 Dorothy E Lindsay, *Report upon a study of the Diet of the Labouring Classes in Glasgow: carried out during 1911–1913 under the auspices of the Corporation of the City* (Glasgow, 1913), pp.23–24.
61 Lloyd P Gartner, *op.cit.,*pp.150–151.
62 *Report on the Physical Condition of Fourteen Hundred Schoolchildren in the City*, City of Edinburgh Charity Organisation Society (London,1906).
63 Anne Hardy, *Epidemic Streets: Infectious Disease and the Rise of Preventive Medicine 1856–1900* (1993), p.288.
64 Dorothy Lindsay, *op.cit.*, p.23.

CHAPTER THREE

Welfare

'. . . no synagogue on the South Side did in any way shirk their respective responsibilities . . . whereas the Garnethill Synagogue had all the time turned a deaf ear to the pitiful cries and shrieks of many poor and unfortunate parents and children . . .'

N. Nathan, Hon. Secretary, Glasgow United Shechita Fund, letter in *Jewish Chronicle*, 25/11/1910

With the continuing movement of impoverished Jews from Eastern Europe to Glasgow, the Jewish community expanded and developed its network of support for its weakest members. This provided welcome and needed relief and offered an alternative both to the rudimentary statutory services, which must have seemed strange and unfamiliar to the alien newcomers, and to the comparatively well-financed and pervasive evangelical Christian missionary facilities.

The Jewish leadership had their own reasons for involvement in charitable activities besides the clear benefits it provided for their poorer co-religionists. They felt the need to engage in philanthropic work as this was an activity highly prized in Victorian Glasgow. Also, by providing an alternative to the statutory parochial relief and emphasising the deserving nature of the Jewish poor, for example their 'lack of drunkenness',[1] they elevated the status of the Jewish community as one which cared for its own needs, and was therefore worthy of emancipation. There may also have been indirect pressure from the wider community to see Jewish welfare established on a similar basis to its own.[2]

Support, however, was not be doled out on an indiscriminate basis. Care was taken to ensure that the poor were really deserving, enabling the communal leadership to retain the power of patronage over the newer arrivals. Visitors from the Glasgow Hebrew Philanthropic Society made sure that the poor would spend grants appropriately and that they led a 'respectable' way of life.[3] While charity in Hebrew is rendered as *tzedaka*, which has connotations of 'right-doing', in Glasgow, as in most other contemporary British communities, charity was not seen as an end in itself, which might pauperise the recipient and create a culture of dependency, but rather as a means of curing poverty by encouraging economic development.[4]

Self-sufficiency was also encouraged by grants to employers to take on immigrant workers during their first weeks of work.[5] These philanthropic aims achieved some degree of success. Funds were raised in the 1870s, even before the main era of immigration, not just for Jewish relief activities; they were also collected for the city's main hospitals, the Western Infirmary and the Royal Infirmary. This helped to forge good links with the wider community, while covering the costs of hospitalisation of poor Jews. The various fledgling Jewish welfare organisations formed during the period of mass immigration eventually provided a bewildering choice of potential support for the poor. However, they could not compare with the experience or the strength of the Glasgow Jewish Board of Guardians. This body's origins can be dated back at least to the 1840s as during the synagogal schism of the time there was at least one Jewish welfare body in existence.[6] This probably paralleled the formation of the Edinburgh Hebrew Philanthropic Benefit Society in 1838 as it is unlikely that Glasgow Jewry would not have emulated the Edinburgh community in providing for the needs of their poorer members.[7] Similar bodies were also established in Liverpool in 1808 and Manchester in 1825 and these may have served as the model for later developments.

For many years Jewish charity in Glasgow was run by the synagogue, and the Glasgow Hebrew Philanthropic Society was certainly in existence before the opening of the George Street Synagogue in 1858. At this time the Society had its own committee and the services of Asher Asher, newly qualified in medicine, the first Glasgow Jew to do so, as its medical officer.[8] Both the synagogue executive, who disbursed congregational charitable funds, and the Philanthropic Society were called on regularly, from as early as the 1860s, to disburse some of their limited resources to assist transmigrants to continue with their journey westwards.[9] This aid was aimed to prevent a substantial increase in the numbers of destitute newcomers arriving in Glasgow, with its potential social and economic consequences, although it might have had the opposite effect of attracting newcomers to the city.

In 1876 Jewish welfare in Glasgow ceased to be the daily responsibility of the synagogue executive when the charitable work of the synagogue was formally integrated into the activities of the Philanthropic Society.[10] This mirrored developments in London where the formation of the London Jewish Board of Guardians in 1859 reflected the secularisation of communal philanthropy, forming an organisation intended to apply its aid more rationally and in a form preferred by the wider society.[11] The welfare activities still carried a medical dimension with various doctors employed to provide treatment for the Jewish poor. A number of non-Jewish doctors, Paterson, Pinkerton, Middleton and Morton, continued the work established by Asher Asher. Doctors were engaged at an honorarium of 5 guineas a year with 10/- extra paid for a confinement. A pharmacist called Grieg supplied medicines at cost.[12] Alfred Finkelstein, appointed at the end of the nineteenth century, was only the second Jewish medical officer of the Society.[13]

Many of the welfare cases dealt with by the Philanthropic Society during 1879 were living in such Gorbals streets as Thistle Street and Portugal Street, reflecting the changing geographic balance of the community from north to south of the River Clyde. Dr. Middleton had to resign his post as Medical Officer of the Glasgow Hebrew Philanthropic Society in 1881 because the Society's clientele were mainly resident south of the river and the extra travelling time involved meant that he could not do justice to the main parts of his work.[14] The appointment in

October 1881 of Dr. Morton, who lived at 55 Dixon Avenue, in the Crosshill area a mile to the south of the Gorbals, is a further confirmation of this population shift. Morton had a surgery at 90 Main Street in the Gorbals and the financial arrangement with the Philanthropic Society gave him 2/- for each house call and 1/- for each consultation at the surgery.[15]

From 1886 it was clear that the Hebrew Philanthropic Society, created to care for the resident poor of a much smaller community, was finding it hard to cope with the many new demands for welfare relief, even in its new role, from 1890, as the Glasgow Jewish Board of Guardians. Usually led by a successful Garnethill businessman, its income and its expenditure grew considerably during the Presidency of David Heilbron, a Glasgow wine merchant with other financial interests, particularly in the theatre. From about £200 in 1878 expenditure reached £348 in 1886 due to the needs of an increasing number 'of foreign poor'.[16]

The expenditure of the Glasgow Jewish Board of Guardians was a barometer of the situation in the wider Jewish world. Deteriorating conditions in Russia left communities disrupted with thousands of destitute Jews on the move. The community responded with a rapid growth in welfare activities in the 1890s followed by a period of consolidation. Between 1891 and 1892 the number of welfare cases handled by the Jewish Board of Guardians increased by no less than one-third and the Board were forced to seek financial aid from the Russian Jewish Relief Fund in London.[17] After 1892 the pace of Jewish immigration slowed a little and travellers arriving in Edinburgh were said to be less destitute, possibly because the price of travel meant that poorer Jews could not afford to get to America. Some Jews from Moscow settling in Scotland were said to be well educated and to have some funds with them.[18] Nevertheless, extra costs were still falling on local Jewish welfare bodies.

In 1898 the Board of Guardians spent £523 on 385 relief cases.[19] About five years later in 1903 the Board of Guardians could report that they had helped over 341 cases at a reduced cost of £346.10.0. While some of the money was used for training and industrial rehabilitation, most of the funds were spent in direct relief.[20] The sum of £47, more than 13% of relief funding, was allocated for train and steamer fares as the Board attempted to reunite families. A number of individuals were enabled to return, or were 'repatriated' to families on the Continent or in Russia, and some wives and children were assisted to join the head of the household who had preceded them, usually to the United States.[21]

Fundraising in Glasgow thus had to deal with the dual needs of the increasing numbers of the local Jewish poor as well as for general relief for Russian Jewry. For this there was much support in Glasgow, and public expression came in June 1891 with a civic meeting convened by Lord Provost John Muir at the request of Sir John Cuthbertson and a group of Christian ministers.[22] The Lord Provost said that he had no wish to offend the Russian Government, though the meeting, expressing much pro-Jewish sentiment, called on the British Government to intervene to ameliorate the Jewish suffering in Russia.[23] This political meeting was followed by major civic fundraising in April 1892 when a Glasgow-wide initiative, complementing similar moves in other major British cities, raised over £2,432.[24]

Glasgow Jewry organised its own fund-raising to supplement the funds collected by the city. The Jewish Board of Guardians launched a special appeal for additional subscriptions and in December 1891 put on a concert in the St. Andrew's Halls, near the Garnethill Synagogue, which was filled with members of the community.[25] The Jewish friendly society, the Court 'Sons of Isaac', also organised a concert.[26] Despite all these efforts subsidies still had to be provided by the Russo-Jewish Relief Fund from London. To cope with the growing community during the years before the First World War a number of new Jewish social and welfare agencies came into being and some older organisations entered a period of consolidation. The first attempts at institutional care commenced during this period and the organisations providing Jewish relief all came to be centred in the Gorbals where most of their clientele were to be found. New friendly societies continued to be formed and the existing groups grew and widened the scope of their activities. This left the Board of Guardians with the role of concentrating their aid on the most needy, that is those unable to create their own networks of self-help.

The Board of Guardians underpinned their new increased responsibilities with regular, major fundraising initiatives. They were supported at different times by an Aid Society and an Auxiliary Group of younger fundraisers and had the backing of the Hebrew Ladies' Benevolent Society.[27] In addition, the Theatre Royal regularly gave its premises free for the holding of charity concerts for Jewish causes, under the auspices of the Heilbron family.[28] In 1909 and 1910, charity concerts, in aid of the Jewish poor of Glasgow, were held in the Palace Theatre attended on both occasions by no fewer than 3,000 people.[29]

With the continued expansion in the community more specialist welfare groups were founded. Not all of these were formed in the Gorbals. It was with the aim of targeting the specific needs of the poor and the unemployed that the Glasgow Hebrew Boot, Clothing and Employment Assistance Guild was set up in January 1907, after a meeting at Garnethill.[30] The organisers of the Guild immediately agreed to work with the other Jewish charitable groups in the city to prevent overlap.[31] Soon after the first meeting the Guild was reorganised to take into account the preponderance of Jewish poverty in the Gorbals area, south of the Clyde. During its first year the Guild provided 150 pairs of boots, fifty sets of clothing and found employment for 150 at a cost of £58.[32]

Other welfare societies replicated in the Gorbals the charitable forms familiar to the Jewish newcomers to Glasgow who had originated in the *shtetls* of Eastern Europe. In the early years of the twentieth century Moses Aaron, known affectionately as *Reb Moshe*, founded the *Lechem Aniyim*, literally Bread for the Poor, though usually known in English as the Jewish Distribution Society.[33] This was specifically established to provide the Gorbals poor with bread and other basic foodstuffs. Neither *Reb Moshe* nor his supporters were particularly well off but he managed to obtain remarkable gifts of goods in kind rather than collecting money. In 1913 he collected and distributed 18,350 loaves of bread, 3846 candles, 676 lbs of meat and 670 lbs of sugar. He distributed kosher wine, milk, flour and an item, probably tobacco, which was described as being 'for the comfort of some old men'.[34] The Society was based at South Portland Street Synagogue and was virtually always synonymous with its elderly founder although it continued running into the 1930s with a second collector.[35]

More specifically for young members of the community the Jewish Children's Fresh Air Fund was set up in June 1908 to cater for the religious needs of Jewish children who had previously been taken to holiday homes which were not under Jewish supervision and where kosher food would not be provided.[36] The need for the provision of country holidays for children cooped up in Gorbals streets all year and whose parents were unable to take them on vacation seemed clear to most. There was, however, a small but vocal group who spurned such paternalistic gestures and advocated better living conditions rather than the acceptance of a week's charity in the summer.[37] This Fund proved to be popular and continued to operate until the Second World War, run by the Boot and Clothing Fund, with financial support from the Glasgow Corporation Education Department.[38]

With the proliferation of new charities there was always concern at the Board of Guardians that the competition would affect their income and they were particularly concerned about private charitable efforts aimed at relieving the needs of just one person or one family. The Board felt that such activities, while obviously motivated by a desire to help the neediest members of the community, detracted from their attempts to conduct a community-based strategy for welfare provision both for charitable collections and for the implementation of policy. There was a little of the north-south divide involved as the Board pointed out that such collections were invariably taking place on the South Side.[39] In addition, the Board felt the need to ensure that applicants were deserving of relief, and with increasing numbers of the community depending on weekly payments it was necessary to be careful with communal funds.

A frequent complaint of the Board was their belief that other

Jewish communities in Scotland sent casual applicants for relief through to Glasgow.[40] By 1907 the Board's expenditure exceeded £1,157 annually and 1193 cases were supported.[41] The next year saw pressures mount on the Board. Expenditure fell to £857 but there were 1,500 applications for assistance and relief operations had to be suspended for three months. In January 1910 Michael Simons, concerned about the emphasis of Jewish fundraising, expressed the opinion that

> . . . the efforts put forward by the Zionists in the furtherance of their movement might be partly concentrated on the relief of the Jewish poor. A reasonable share of the relief of the poor was not borne by every Jew in Glasgow.[42]

Unfortunately, there was little change in the situation over the next few years and even in 1913 income was only £785. Fundraising activities were stepped up, even involving the civic authorities in Jewish charitable functions. A Charity Ball in January 1913 at the Grosvenor, under the patronage of the Lord Provost and city magistrates, made a profit of £85.[43]

Until 1911 the work of the Jewish Board of Guardians had been conducted from the synagogue chambers in Garnethill. It had been clear for some time that this arrangement was quite unsatisfactory, given that the recipients of relief were mainly to be found in the Gorbals. However, communal leaders at Garnethill, following the break-up of the United Synagogue which had given them control over the Gorbals synagogues, feared that moving premises to the Gorbals would remove their leadership in communal philanthropy.[44] As time went by the needs to have premises in the Gorbals, which would also function as a welfare centre, increased considerably. As a first step Daniel Rosenbloom, Chairman of the Strangers' Aid Society, agreed to form a support committee for the Board of Guardians on the South Side in September 1907 but the need for a physical presence in the Gorbals eventually became overwhelming.[45] At the AGM of the Board of Guardians in February 1911 the decision to move to new rented headquarters at 11 Apsley Place was confirmed.[46]

The acceptance by Garnethill of the need for the key Jewish welfare body to be based in the Gorbals confirmed the inevitability of the passage of communal authority from north to south. Garnethill bodies were slow to affiliate to the Gorbals-based Glasgow Jewish Representative Council when it was formed in 1914 but there was no alternative to joining on the same terms as for other communal organisations. However, Garnethill's leading role was still regularly acknowledged and communal deputations were likely to be made up of leading members of both Garnethill and the Representative Council.[47] This is not to say that there was no tension between the two groups. Resentment over Garnethill's alleged financial oppression of the Gorbals poor spilled over in November 1910 when the Secretary of the United Shechita Fund accused Garnethill, in a letter to the *Jewish Chronicle*, of using revenue from the sale of kosher meat in the Gorbals to subsidise the synagogue at the expense of the bereaved poor. Gorbals poor were usually supported by similar revenue obtained from the locally based *shechita* bodies, in competition with Garnethill:

> . . . no synagogue on the South Side did in any way shirk their respective responsibilities . . . whereas the Garnethill Synagogue had all the time turned a deaf ear to the pitiful cries and shrieks of many poor and unfortunate parents and children . . .[48]

It was hoped that the concentration of Jewish welfare resources in one building would lead to better co-ordination of activities with the other Jewish welfare groups. The Board of Guardians expected that working closely together would prevent duplication of effort by permitting access to the financial records of all the various Jewish welfare groups. A further evident need was some professionalisation of the welfare services as voluntary establishment figures could not continue to provide the day-to-day requirements in rota relief. This mirrored developments in mainstream charitable bodies.[49]

Despite the move to the Gorbals the Board of Guardians remained, under the Presidency of Michael Simons, essentially a Garnethill organisation. The office-bearers in 1913 were all members of the Garnethill Synagogue with the only South Side executive officer being Ellis Isaacs, who was one of the six Vice-Presidents.[50] The council also showed the same preponderance, with only one South Sider, Barnet Lipschitz, among its twelve members. Ellis Isaacs and Barnet Lipschitz both had a long history of communal service and it was possibly not surprising that the increasingly large community in the Gorbals and beyond felt the need to add locally based and run welfare groups that would be seen to be more responsive to their needs. Writing of the Glasgow Jewish Board of Guardians in the period after the First World War, Benjamin described the receipt of rota relief as a brutalising experience:

> The humiliating atmosphere in which items of clothing were dispensed was quite Dickensian . . . having to declare one's poverty to a panel of austere patronising individuals . . .[51]

In the troubled conditions of the time it was not only with the other communal charity organisations that the Board of Guardians had to co-ordinate activities. The Board were dealing with a number of cases of deserted wives whose husbands were said to have gone on to the United States, and the United Hebrew Charities of New York were helpful in supplying information.[52] The costs of running the facilities at 11 Apsley Place were heavy, with the first year's expenses being about £131. Questions were asked about the Board's level of organisational and administration expenses but the President, Michael Simons, was at pains to point out at the AGM in February 1912 that these compared favourably with other similar charities and referred to the need to make investigations to ensure the genuineness of prospective claimants.

Glasgow, which now had the fourth largest Jewish community in Britain after London, Manchester and Leeds, was found, in a major regional survey carried out in 1906 of Jewish relief work in Britain, to have one of the lowest levels of per capita charitable contributions in the country.[53] By 1906 a substantial national Jewish welfare network had been established in Britain but there were wide discrepancies between the charitable contributions of the different communities.[54] In Glasgow only 2/8d. was collected annually by the main Jewish charities, which compared with Birmingham, the highest at 11/- per head, and Edinburgh at 3/10d. The survey could obtain no clear reason for these wide discrepancies. A higher figure might represent a higher level of poverty, either of native or transient Jews, or even denote a community with a higher capability for raising money for welfare relief. Nationally throughout the United Kingdom, with a population of 42 million, poor relief cost £16 million, or about 7/7d. per head so that the amounts collected within the Jewish community can be seen as a substantial charge on its resources. Most communities surveyed in the report had a free loan society, similar to the Hebrew Benevolent Loan Society in Glasgow, which compared favourably, both with the number of loans granted and the sums advanced, with similar bodies round the country.[55]

One of the conclusions of the survey was the need for the larger communities to form their own Central Charitable Board, to co-ordinate relief work and to improve uptake of benefits by those in real need. Within a few weeks of the publication of this report a Glasgow Jewish Charitable Board was formed.[56] This was composed of representatives from the Board of Guardians, Talmud Torah, Strangers' Aid Society and the Jewish Hospital Fund and Sick Visiting Association as well as delegates from the Glasgow synagogues. The committee members of this new grouping were all active in different areas within the community and the committee comprised many of the leaders of Gorbals Jewry. The stimulus to the formation of the Central Charitable Board was not just the article in the *Jewish Chronicle*. With the recent break-up of the United Synagogue there was felt to be a need for community co-ordination to provide for the poor of the community. This had been particularly so with regard to matters which had been dealt with by the United Synagogue such as pauper funerals and the distribution of charitable collections. However, the aims of the Glasgow Jewish Charitable Board were much more modest than proposed in the *Jewish Chronicle*. There was no attempt to co-ordinate welfare policy or activity and the Board merely sought to co-operate in the collection and dispersal of charitable funds made at marriages and other celebrations. Glasgow Jewry's organisations showed again that they could work together in specific areas of mutual self-interest only as long as it did not involve giving up their own areas of independence.

During the First World War there was a continuing need for funds to support Jews in lands of distress abroad such as Serbia, occupied Belgium and Poland. Jews continued to face severe disabilities in Russia, and the Turks were increasingly harassing the nascent Zionist body in Palestine. The continued appeals for Jews abroad, many of them conducted on an emergency *ad hoc* basis, put the Glasgow Jewish Board of Guardians under some pressure and naturally affected their income. In addition, the number of people requiring relief continued to rise, by no less than 35% between 1915 and 1916.[57] The war took many bread-winners to the battlefront and increased the cost of food and clothing. The need for the Jewish community to support the general war effort also meant that human resources for voluntary work were stretched. The founding of the Jewish Central Relief Fund helped in the co-ordination of Jewish activities but the need to cope with general civic problems as well as with increasing Jewish distress at home and abroad inevitably caused it financial difficulties.

Early in the War there had been a depression in the tailoring trade and the Board, requiring an infusion of money from beyond its regular 400 subscribers, had to turn for support to the Union of Jewish Tailors and Pressers, as well as other Jewish trade unions and the Jewish friendly societies, during 1916.[58] This indirect appeal to the Gorbals community through some of its major institutions provided a valuable source of funds which the Board could not reach directly.

Glasgow Jewry showed its ability to assimilate traditional Jewish patterns of philanthropy to those around them in Victorian Scottish society.[59] Charitable endeavour marked out the successful and gave them a key role in voluntary work, and this in turn enhanced their social status. Further, in an age when statutory provision was rudimentary, Glasgow Jews could fall back on patterns of social cohesion learned in Eastern Europe while gaining support from a municipality only too keen to support voluntary activity as a means of reducing the burden on the city rates.[60] With the beginnings of twentieth-century socialist radicalism the Jewish community found that its strengths were based not just within its religious traditions but within a society which possessed a powerful political element where a strong sense of egalitarianism prevailed.

Friendly and Mutual Benefit Societies

The establishment of a network of Jewish friendly societies considerably enhanced the social cohesion of the community, and its welfare provision. These societies enabled their members to provide assistance during illness and support for widows and orphans. Funded by the weekly penny contributions of their members, these societies encouraged self-reliance in the immigrant community. The principle of mutual benefit, once well established in the Jewish branches of the friendly society movement, soon extended into other areas. It was the basis for the formation of such vital community bodies as the Hebrew Benevolent Loan Society (1888), the Glasgow Jewish Naturalisation Society (1902) and the Glasgow Hebrew Burial Society (1907).[61]

The friendly society movement became the most widespread form of association among Jewish workers in Britain, conforming to the general pattern of working-class saving, though not initially covering women or children.[62] The impetus for the formation of these societies matched similar developments in other communities based on the financial advantages of the friendly society movement, guaranteed by the Friendly Societies Act of 1896. By the interwar years, 1918–1939, there were more friendly societies in Glasgow than any other type of Jewish body, including synagogues. Thus the friendly societies could be described as a mass movement of Glasgow Jews rivalling the synagogues, and the burial societies, in their levels of membership. It was important for those Jews who sought an active and involved attachment to

Jewish community institutions yet were unable, sometimes for ideological reasons, to express their attachment through synagogue membership. Not all the immigrants were religious and many did not maintain affiliation to the synagogues. Thus the role of the friendly societies in enhancing the cohesion of the Jewish community, particularly for its more marginal members, was crucial.

What was to become a network of Jewish self-help groups in the Gorbals began as early as 1878 with the formation of a Glasgow Hebrew Sick Society which raised its funds by annual fundraising dinners and balls held in the Standard Halls on Gorbals Main Street. In Manchester, a similarly named society, formed about twenty years earlier, functioned not like the later friendly societies but rather as a contributory insurance society managed by the communal leadership.[63] In Glasgow there is no evidence for this kind of organisation, and the impetus for the Hebrew Sick Society may have come from Isaac Isaacs who had moved from London to Glasgow in about 1870 and brought his friendly society involvement with him.[64] In 1886 Isaacs, helped by another Gorbals Jewish leader, Jacob Samuels, founded the Court 'Sons of Isaac' Friendly Society as a branch of the non-Jewish Order of Foresters. One of the aims of the Society was to support wage-earners during the *shiva*, the formal week of mourning, an inevitable event in Victorian times given the frequency of child deaths and the financial hardship caused by the missing of a week of work.

The Jewish friendly society movement developed rapidly during the 1880s. While the first Jewish societies were affiliated to a number of non-Jewish orders, as the Sons of Isaac had been, gradually Jewish fraternal orders were formed. Glasgow affiliates were added, especially in the first years of the twentieth century.[65] A Jewish Workingmen's Club was founded at 12 Rutherglen Road in the Gorbals in October 1891, setting up a 'friendly section', or *bikur cholim*, which would provide medical care for member families for a weekly subscription of 3d.[66] Friendly societies quickly became popular as the means through which poorer people dealt with financial risks though there was still a stratum of newly arrived immigrants, the irregularly employed and the very poor who could not meet the regular subscriptions demanded.[67] They also proved to be a good investment, providing workers with valuable benefits over a lifetime for the sums expended.[68] The new Glasgow societies, founded in the first years of the twentieth century, were usually affiliated to national Jewish friendly society bodies based in London such as the Grand Order of Israel and the Order Achei Brith and Shield of Abraham. The local societies were organised in Lodges, the first to be set up, in 1903, being the Lord Rothschild No.18 and the Dr. Herzl Lodge, both affiliates of the Grand Order of Israel.

The societies had their own voluntary sick visitor, loan and welfare facilities and often provided their own medical officers. Members could receive financial help and practical assistance in times of distress such as during illness, unemployment and bereavement. During sickness, for example, benefit could be paid for up to about thirteen weeks, with half benefit thereafter, and the costs of all medication covered. It was clearly preferable to use the facilities provided by the friendly society, for which one's subscription provided automatic entitlements, than to turn to the Board of Guardians with its heavy-handed application of rota relief. Indeed, in London the Jewish Board of Guardians considered it a sign of a lack of thrift if applicants for welfare were not members of a friendly society.

Contributions to the different societies varied but usually ranged from 1/3 to 3/- weekly. This implied an annual contribution of at least £3.60 and in some cases up to £7.80. Some maintained membership of more than one society and in the event of problems could be eligible for a variety of benefits. This could enable a subscriber, and his family, to emerge financially unscathed from a significant illness. Medical services were often part of the benefit package with local general practitioners treating enrolled members. Some Gorbals doctors derived much of their income from their position as the medical officer of a friendly society. However, it was sometimes alleged that a friendly society with an official medical officer might end up providing less than ideal medical care and inferior drugs.[69] A sense of complacency, from a position of medical tenure, could lead to abuses in the doctor-patient relationship.

The membership rules of the Lord Rothschild Lodge specified that sick members had to be examined by a doctor with a Gorbals practice and would not receive benefit until the doctor's certificate had reached J Rosenbloom, the Lodge's secretary.[70] The doctor's permission was also required for the patient to leave his home. Indeed, a member could be fined if he was found to be working when he was supposed to be ill at home or when he was seen at 'any place of amusement or at any house but his home'.

These groups served a much-needed social as well as welfare function. With their colourful rituals and uniforms, certificates and sashes, they helped bring some brightness into many otherwise dull lives.[71] The social aspects of some of the societies, such as in the Odessa Lodge, often reflected *landsmanschaft* links fostered by immigrant groups from the same small East European towns, or *shtetls*. Life in the *shtetl* had a certain unchanging character despite the economic privation. The *landsmanshaftn*, particularly strong in the immigrant community in New York, remained religiously traditional, acting as a bulwark against assimilation by promoting the old values, unlike the American Jewish fraternal orders which promoted acculturation.[72]

As we have seen, the main Glasgow lodges were named after major Jewish personalities like Lord Rothschild and Theodore Herzl. Some friendly society names reflected local Jewish dignitaries, like Rabbi Shyne, while others were named after more distant Jewish heroes and heroines like King David and Queen Esther. By 1907 women were beginning to form their own lodges although the main impetus for women's lodges did not come until the Lloyd George National Insurance Act of 1911. From small beginnings the friendly societies remained, certainly until the establishment of the National Health Service in 1949, one of the major elements of Glasgow Jewry.

During these pre-War years the growth of the Jewish friendly societies was quite remarkable. While, as we have seen, most of the lodges were affiliates of the Grand Order of Israel, and of the Achei

Brith and Shield of Abraham, there was one order, the Beacons of the Order of Ancient Maccabeans, which had a strong Zionist orientation, in addition to its friendly society functions. The National Insurance Act of 1911 provided for compulsory insurance of manual workers and lower-paid non-manual workers funded by workers' contributions as well as sums from employers and from the state. Non-naturalised Jews fell outside the full provisions of the Act until it was amended in 1918 to embrace all contributors. In the meantime the state withheld its 2d weekly contribution to resident aliens although it was reckoned that the Jewish friendly societies could cope with the shortfall owing to the better health of its members.[73]

The changes introduced by the Natural Insurance Act had important implications for all the friendly societies, and regular talks, in Yiddish, explaining the changes were given by society leaders to the increasing number who took advantage of the financial security in times of stress that membership could confer. The Grand Order of Israel affiliate Lord Rothschild Lodge No.18 remained the largest of the Jewish friendly societies in Glasgow with a membership of over 200 in 1913 and a capital of £585. It was claimed that even nationally 'few Lodges can show such results'.[74] Lord Rothschild Lodge's financial strength enabled it to provide sick pay at the rate of 18/- weekly. However, even with this level of funding the Lodge could not compete with the resources of the Board of Guardians or match its work with the uninsured poor. It was the Lord Rothschild Lodge which took the initiative in Glasgow in making protests to Sir Edward Grey, the Foreign Secretary, over the problems some naturalised Glasgow Jews, in common with Jews from other parts of Britain, were having when trying to enter Russia to visit family while using British passports.[75]

Better provision for women followed the National Insurance Act. The Lord Rothschild Lodge No. 18 agreed to form a ladies' branch after a mass meeting in the Gorbals in January 1913 and the Lady Rothschild Lodge No. 67 was duly inaugurated in June of that year.[76] The Lady Rothschild Lodge quickly organised social functions as well as the normal insurance and welfare activities. A dance held in Diamond's Hall in South Portland Street in October 1913 was much appreciated since '. . . functions were looked forward to with much interest and help to brighten an hour or an evening of many persons who would otherwise never know the joy of change from the dull, drab life of the factory'.[77]

Other Grand Order of Israel Lodges in Glasgow included the Dr. Herzl Lodge which had a capital of £359 in 1913, and two further Lodges were established before the War, namely the Dr Adler Lodge, which began with 110 members, and the Rabbi Shyne Lodge, which immediately attracted eighty-five members including Rabbi Hillman, the communal rabbi of Gorbals Jewry. The fact that some ladies from the Lady Rothschild Lodge were present at the inauguration of this Lodge in December 1913 was described as 'a novel feature'.[78] The Achei Brith and Shield of Abraham Lodges tended to be smaller. The leading Glasgow affiliate was the Michael Simons Lodge No. 28, and two new Lodges were opened in 1914. These were the Rev. I. Levine Lodge and the Rev. Eleazar P. Phillips Lodge No. 75 which was aimed at workers and small businessmen. Because of their association with the Garnethill ministers it was hoped to bring members of the community from north and south of the river closer together.[79]

Other societies followed the friendly society model of mutual aid and regular saving. One was the Glasgow Jewish Naturalisation Society, sponsored by the Dr. Herzl Lodge and its indefatigable secretary, Bernard Glasser.[80] With national insurance benefits partially linked to British citizenship, the friendly society movement was an obvious vehicle for encouraging naturalisation. The costs of naturalisation had been put at over £5 and it was clearly easier for those taking this path to save regularly, usually at the rate of 1/- per week. The Glasgow Jewish Naturalisation Society came into being after a public meeting held at South Portland Street Synagogue addressed by its founder and first chairman, Jacob Kramrisch. Kramrisch recognised that, besides any financial benefits, the Jewish newcomers would not feel part of the society in which they lived without achieving citizenship, and the low uptake of British nationality by Gorbals Jewry can be confirmed by the presence of very few Jewish names on the Gorbals voters' roll. Within a few months the Naturalisation Society had collected over £41, and by the end of the first year five out of the thirty-five members had been successful in obtaining British nationality.[81] Actually, the Society's advertising referred to becoming 'English' citizens as it took another generation before the concept of being Scottish was widely understood.

Another major society encouraging saving and mutual aid was the Glasgow Hebrew Burial Society, founded in 1907 in response to the major challenge of providing affordable funerals in an age when funerals of children and young adults were only too frequent. With burial grounds at Sandymount and eventually at Glenduffhill in the east end of Glasgow, the Burial Society still provides its services to members on a mutual aid basis free at the point of need.

Although the Jewish Board of Guardians set aside a sum of money annually for cash loans, it was the Glasgow Hebrew Benevolent Loan Society, founded in 1888, which specialised in the provision of interest-free loans to members of the community.[82] The Glasgow society functioned as a mutual aid society with subscribers joining it as a 'penny society', paying 1d for their weekly 'share'. This principle was clearly now well established within Glasgow Jewry. Benevolent Society loans were extended to those who required temporary financial assistance or who were looking for aid in becoming financially independent. This was a common type of Jewish charitable endeavour in the areas where the new immigrants settled, and similar enterprises were formed in Edinburgh and Dundee. It was moreover a form of aid, not found in society at large, which grew directly out of Jewish religious principles of preventing poverty rather than merely giving relief. The Loan Society seems to have grown out of the activities of a small welfare group seeking to provide blankets and coal for the needy.[83] Within a year the Society had 300 subscribers raising about £65 annually.[84] The income from shares was augmented by the repayment of loans and by larger donations. However, for many years it was the penny subscriptions that funded the bulk of the Society's activities.

The beginnings of the Loan Society illustrate the quick response both by the newcomers themselves and the Garnethill leadership to the requirements of the time. Very quickly a series of mutual aid societies and welfare systems were organised, and this showed the ability of Scottish Jewry to establish organisations capable of dealing with the needs of its weaker members. They underlined the determination of the Jews to defend their community and improve its status. In addition to the purely welfare considerations this aided the cohesion of the community and promoted the idea in the wider community that the Jews looked after the needs of their own needy co-religionists. The Jews of Glasgow clearly demonstrated during this immigrant period that they could be examples of self-help and assertiveness.

Residential Care

REFUGE HOSTEL: There was little in the way of residential care within the Glasgow Jewish community in the pre-1919 period as Glasgow's Jews were not sufficiently numerous to justify the provision of a hospital. The first residential establishment was the refuge hostel set up by the Jewish Strangers Aid (*Hachnasat Orchim*) Society in the Gorbals in May 1897 to provide accommodation and welfare for Jewish travellers just arrived in the city.[85] Onward travellers, awaiting the trans-Atlantic crossing, had usually been accommodated in a number of different hostels within the city with an overflow in private homes.[86] There was often a concern about the health of these transmigrants, such as at the time of a cholera scare in Glasgow in 1893.[87] At the same time an outbreak of cholera in Russia caused such concern about the number of travellers from Russia passing through Glasgow that a special sanitary inspector was appointed to keep watch on those lodging houses frequented by the transmigrants. Lodging houses, always a potent source of spread of infection, were also a target for local health officials during recurrent smallpox outbreaks during the 1890s.

Given these health problems, the opening of a Jewish refuge hostel, albeit on a small scale, must have been some help in controlling the risks of infection and in providing reliable hospitality for short-term accommodation. The Jewish community in Edinburgh established a similar hostel, the House of Refuge, at the beginning of the twentieth century. This was modelled on the London Poor Jews' Temporary Shelter. This Shelter had been crucial not only in providing short-term accommodation, but had ensured safety for the newcomers at the docks where by employing an interpreter and retired policemen they prevented the migrants being tricked and robbed.[88] The Glasgow Jewish Refuge accommodated about 200 people for short stays in 1904, usually of about a week, until they could make more definite arrangements, whether for local residence or for onward travel. By 1906 the numbers accommodated had reached 400 and the annual costs had increased from £77 to £112.[89] However, after the passage of the Aliens Act, and the requirement for arrivals to have at least £5, the need for a refuge hostel gradually decreased and it closed around 1910 or 1911.

ORPHANAGE: The care of orphaned children had posed a problem for many years, given the number of premature deaths of tuberculosis sufferers and the families who had become divided during the period of immigration. Though extended family links were strong, there were many who had no obvious support, and by 1913 the need for a Jewish orphanage was clear. The Merryflatts Poorhouse in Govan, then a separate burgh adjacent to Glasgow, had a number of Jewish men, women and also young children in its care from the 1890s although the numbers were never very large. In 1908 only seventy-five Jews were receiving poor relief in all of Scotland, fifty-three in Govan and twelve in Glasgow.[90]

The decision to consider opening a Jewish orphanage in Glasgow was taken in February 1913 to care for Jewish orphans and deserted children then looked after by local authorities in the parishes of Glasgow and Govan.[91] Support was promised by members of the parish councils of up to £100, which was about one third of the anticipated annual costs. Conditional support was given by Rabbi Hillman provided that the children admitted were halachically Jewish. The financial burden of establishing the orphanage was eased by the offer, from Joseph Jacobson, to provide the necessary building in memory of his daughter Gertrude. A circular was prepared, signed by local Rabbis and ministers, appealing for financial support to let the project begin. By May 1913, following a report by Rev. E.P. Phillips, for many years the President of the orphanage, on the progress of the provisional committee, the decision was taken to proceed with the opening.[92]

In June 1913 the Gertrude Jacobson Orphanage was inaugurated in a stone semi-detached house at 53 Millbrae Road, in the Battlefield area near both the Queens Park Synagogue and the Victoria Infirmary. The first children were admitted in time for the official opening in November 1913 which was carried out by Michael Simons and Rev. E.P. Phillips.[93] The accommodation in Millbrae Road extended to seven rooms, and while it was estimated that sixteen children could be housed there, it was decided to start with about ten children, representing four families. J. Mitchell of Govan Parish and J.R. Motion of Glasgow attended the opening and pledged their support although they felt that the home was operating at about capacity. They advised that if there was to be expansion, then another home should be purchased.

The Orphanage managed to operate successfully during the war years with about ten orphans in care. With the end of the war there were additional pressures with new Jewish refugees and an increased number of orphaned children. An appeal was launched, quickly raising £500, to obtain and endow a larger building.[94] The Edinburgh community set up a committee to aid with fundraising and organised summer holidays for current residents in Portobello. The new orphanage at 6 Sinclair Drive, not far from the original building, had accommodation for up to forty children and was surrounded by spacious gardens, including an orchard. During the war about ten refugee children from Belgium were cared for and in October 1920 a group of ten Hungarian children were accommodated.[95] Rev. Phillips maintained a long and close association with the children, and those involved in running the orphanage, Miss Samuels and the Lubins, created a warm and harmonious environment. Jack Cowen, resident from the opening in 1913, recollected that 'it wasn't an orphanage, it was a home, and we were treated with respect wherever we went, because we were from Gertrude Jacobson, and I shall never forget it'.[96]

OLD AGE HOME: About the time the orphanage was opened, the need for some provision of residential care for the Jewish elderly in the Gorbals was also identified. While naturally it was felt to be important to provide a Jewish alternative for those older members of the community living in the Poorhouse, this formed less of a priority than the needs of orphaned Jewish children. Rabbi Katz, of the Queens Park Synagogue, and Rabbi Mendelsohn, of the Oxford Street Synagogue, called a meeting in January 1909 and this led to the formation of a committee and a call for prospective applicants.[97] Katz was elected President but nothing more is heard about this committee until representatives of the Old Age Home committee and the Strangers' Aid Society held a 'conference' about eighteen months later.[98]

With the decline in demand for the Strangers' Aid Society's Refuge the provision of institutional care for the elderly would have seemed a suitable new area for their committee to tackle. Again little action was taken after this conference in September 1910 until a third meeting was convened at South Portland Street Synagogue by Lazarus Ognall, Vice-President of the original committee, in July 1913 to reconsider the possibility of a Jewish old age home.[99] It was realised that there would be competition with the orphanage for financial support and that there was some feeling in the community that there were too many new charities. It was felt that they should delay making a final decision as it would be 'regrettable, if when once opened the Home was compelled to close for lack of funds'.

Just a week later a decision on a home for the elderly was taken.[100] The proposal was for a very small institution beginning with only two or three residents. A sale of work had yielded enough funds to rent accommodation in the Gorbals for a year and some furnishings had been promised by some 'generous sympathisers'.

The principal method of funding was to be by penny subscriptions and it was hoped that if 600 supporters could be enrolled and given some donations in kind, the costs could be met. To try and attract subscribers it was proposed that residents would perform some minor religious services in return for their board and keep:

> male inmates will attend for *minyan* at houses of subscribers during *shiva* and one of the inmates will attend the synagogue to recite the *kaddish* for deceased subscribers during the year following death and on each anniversary.[101]

By September 1913, while the full target of 600 subscribers had not been reached, the committee were encouraged by the support received and proceeded to rent a flat at 3 Nicolson Street in the Gorbals.[102] Although the orphaned children were being accommodated in the more prosperous Langside area, it seemed more suitable for the elderly to be located in an area with which they were more familiar and which had a more intensive Jewish life. It was to be a couple of months before the committee were confident enough to admit the first resident out of a number of applicants. However, the home was finally ready for the official opening which was carried out by Michael Simons just one week after he formally opened the orphanage.[103] Simons referred to the small scale of the Jewish Shelter and Home for Aged Jews, commended Lazarus Ognall and Ellis Isaacs for their efforts and trusted that a larger scheme might come to fruition in the future.

The functioning of the new home remained precarious though Ognall reported a lack of voluntary helpers rather than a shortage of funds early in 1914. Unfortunately, Ognall died in May 1917 and there is no record of the Home after his death. It was to take some considerable time to establish a Jewish old age home in Glasgow. A house at 61 Dixon Avenue, in the Crosshill area, was purchased for use as a Jewish old age home in 1929 but the project did not come to fruition and the house was subsequently used as a synagogue. It was not until 1949 that a Jewish residential home for the elderly in Scotland was set up, in Newark Drive in the Pollokshields area of Glasgow.

CONVALESCENT HOME: By the end of the First World War there was a definite trend within the national friendly society movement for the provision of nursing and convalescent homes.[104] By 1919 there were more than twenty Jewish friendly societies in Glasgow and Edinburgh and this gave them the encouragement to undertake the ambitious project of opening a convalescent home, possibly aimed at members returning from sanatoria after treatment for tuberculosis. Binniehall House, near Slammanan in Stirlingshire, and convenient to both Glasgow and Edinburgh, was opened in April 1921 and the friendly societies were supported in the project by the Glasgow Jewish Hospital and Sick Visiting Society.[105] However, the home was expensive to maintain and it survived barely four years when funding difficulties forced its closure.

References

1 *North British Daily Mail*, 20/6/1891.
2 Rainer Liedtke, *Jewish Welfare in Hamburg and Manchester c1850–1914* (Oxford,1998), pp.75–76.
3 Minutes of the Glasgow Hebrew Philanthropic Society, 30/6/1874, SJAC.
4 Eugene C Black, *The Social Politics of Anglo-Jewry 1880–1920* (Oxford,1988), p.93.
5 Ben Braber, Integration of Jewish Immigrants in Glasgow 1880–1939, unpublished PhD thesis, University of Glasgow, p.212.
6 Kenneth Collins, *Second City Jewry: the Jews of Glasgow in the Age of Expansion 1790–1919* (Glasgow,1990), p.22.
7 Cecil Roth, *The Rise of Provincial Jewry: the Early History of the Jewish Communities in the English Countryside, 1740–1840* (London, 1950), p.59.
8 Kenneth Collins, *op.cit.*, p.25.
9 *Ibid.*, pp.34–35.
10 Minutes of the Glasgow Hebrew Congregation, 25/4/1875, at SJAC.
11 Mordechai Rozin, *The Rich and the Poor: Jewish Philanthropy and Social Control in Nineteenth Century London* (Brighton,1999), p.45.
12 Minutes of the Glasgow Hebrew Philanthropic Society, 1875–1881. Dr.Pinkerton's appointment is confirmed on 18/2/1877.
13 Kenneth Collins, *op.cit.*, p.69.
14 Glasgow Hebrew Philanthropic Society Minutes, 29/5/1881, at SJAC.
15 Ibid., 14/8/1881.
16 *Jewish Chronicle*, 26/11/1886. This compared with an expenditure in Manchester of £1,028 in 1881–1882.
17 *Jewish Chronicle*, 21/10/1892.
18 *Jewish Chronicle*, 9/6/1893.
19 *Jewish Chronicle*, 9/12/1898.
20 *Jewish Chronicle*, 16/1/1903.
21 Kenneth Collins, *op.cit.*, p.106.

22 *Glasgow Herald*, 11/6/1891 and 13/6/1891.
23 *Glasgow Herald*, 15/6/1891.
24 Kenneth Collins, *op.cit.*, p.67.
25 *Jewish Chronicle*, 11/12/1891.
26 *Jewish Chronicle*, 1/4/1892.
27 *Jewish Chronicle*, 18/9/1891.
28 *Jewish Chronicle*, 3/3/1905.
29 *Jewish Chronicle*, 19/2/1909.
30 *Jewish Chronicle*, 4/1/1907.
31 *Jewish Chronicle*, 18/1/1907.
32 *Jewish Chronicle*, 3/1/1908.
33 *Jewish Chronicle*, 19/6/1914.
34 *Jewish Chronicle*, 14/2/1913.
35 Kenneth Collins, *op.cit.*, p.156.
36 *Jewish Chronicle*, 12/6/1908.
37 Ralph Glasser, *Growing up in the Gorbals* (London, 1986), pp.54–55.
38 Kenneth Collins, 'The Growth and Development of Scottish Jewry', in Kenneth Collins, ed., *Aspects of Scottish Jewry* (Glasgow, 1987), p.34.
39 *Jewish Chronicle*, 15/10/1909.
40 *Jewish Chronicle*, 24/3/1911.
41 Annual Reports of the Glasgow Jewish Board of Guardians, SJAC. For Reports before 1912, see *Jewish Chronicle*.
42 *Jewish Chronicle*, 21/1/1910.
43 *Jewish Chron*icle, 3/1/1913.
44 Ben Braber, *op.cit.*, p.212; Eugene C Black, *op.cit.*, p.99.
45 *Jewish Chronicle*, 27/9/1907.
46 *Jewish Chronicle*, 3/2/1911.
47 *Jewish Chronicle*, 21/8/1914, 11/9/1914.
48 Ben Braber, *op.cit.*, p.212; Callum G Brown, *Social History of Religion in Scotland* (London,1987), pp.198–201.
49 *Jewish Chronicle*, 25/11/1910.
50 Annual Report for 1912, Glasgow Jewish Board of Guardians (SJAC).
51 Albert Benjamin, 'The Old Concept of Jewish Welfare', *Jewish Echo*, 27/5/1988, SJAC.
52 *Jewish Chronicle*, 9/2/1912.
53 S. Rosenbloom, 'Jewish Charitable Relief in the Provinces', *Jewish Chronicle*, 14/9/1906, pp.26–27.
54 *Ibid.*,p.26.
55 *Ibid.*,p.27.
56 *Jewish Chronicle*, 30/11/1906.
57 Annual Report, 1915–1916, Glasgow Jewish Board of Guardians, SJAC.
58 *Jewish Chronicle*, 4/2/1916.
59 Olive Checkland, *Philanthropy in Victorian Scotland: Social Welfare and the Voluntary Principle* (Edinburgh,1980), p.31.
60 *Ibid.*, p.311.
61 Report on the foundation of the Glasgow Jewish Naturalisation Society, in Jewish Chronicle, 14/2/1902.
62 David Feldman, *Englishmen and Jews: Social Relations and Political Culture: 1840–1914* (New Haven), p.385.

63 Bill Williams, *The Making of Manchester Jewry 1740–1875* (Manchester, 1985), p.278.
64 *Jewish Chronicle*, 29/1/1897.
65 Kenneth Collins, *Second City Jewry,* p.160.
66 *Jewish Chronicle*, 23/10/1891.
67 Eugene C Black, *op.cit.*, p.196.
68 *Jewish Chronicle*, 8/9/1905.
69 *Jewish Chronicle*, 10/5/1911; Gerry Black, Health and Medical Care of the Jewish Poor in the East End of London: 1880–1939, unpublished PhD thesis, University of Leicester, pp.91–92.
70 Ben Braber, *op.cit.*, p.215.
71 Kenneth Collins, *op.cit.*, p64.
72 Michael R Weisser, *A Brotherhood of Memory: Jewish Landsmanshaftn in the New World* (New York,1985), p.75.
73 Eugene C Black, *op.cit.*, pp.195; Gerry Black, Health and Medical Care of the Jewish Poor in the East End of London, 1880–1939, unpublished PhD thesis, University of Leicester, 1987, p.93.
74 *Jewish Chronicle*, 13/2/1914.
75 *Jewish Chronicle*, 31/1/1913.
76 *Jewish Chronicle*, 3/1/1913; 20/6/1913.
77 *Jewish Chronicle*, 3/10/1913.
78 *Jewish Chronicle*, 26/12/1913.
79 *Jewish Chronicle*, 26/12/1913.
80 *Yiddishe Vanen Tsaitung*, Glasgow, 30/8/1914. A copy of an advertisement for the Glasgow Jewish Naturalisation Society is reproduced in Kenneth Collins, ed., *Aspects of Scottish Jewry* (Glasgow, 1987), p.117.
81 *Jewish Chronicle*, 14/2/1902.
82 Kenneth Collins, *Second City Jewry: the Jews of Glasgow in the Age of Expansion 1790–1919* (Glasgow, 1990), p.67.
83 *Jewish Echo*, 16/3/1928.
84 *Jewish Chronicle*, 23/10/1891.
85 *Jewish Chronicle*, 7/5/1897.
86 Reports of the Glasgow Sanitary Department 1906–1914, Glasgow City Archives, Mitchell Library.
87 Edna Robertson, *Glasgow's Doctor: James Burn Russell 1837–1904* (East Linton, 1998), p.149.
88 Lloyd P. Gartner, *The Jewish Immigrant in England 1870–1914* (London, 1973), p.37.
89 *Jewish Chronicle*, 27/6/1906.
90 *Jewish Chronicle*, 5/6/1908.
91 *Jewish Chronicle*, 14/2/1913.
92 *Jewish Chronicle,* 9/5/1913.
93 *Jewish Chronicle*, 14/11/1913.
94 *Jewish Chronicle*, 5/7/1918.
95 Kenneth Collins, *op.cit.*, p.218.
96 Jack Cowen, recollections of the first years of the Gertrude Jacobson Orphanage, 24/9/1995, in SJAC.
97 *Jewish Chronicle*, 15/1/1909.
98 *Jewish Chronicle*, 2/9/1910.

99 *Jewish Chronicle*, 11/7/1913.
100 *Jewish Chronicle*, 18/7/1913.
101 Kenneth Collins, *op.cit.*, p.163.
102 *Jewish Chronicle*, 12/9/1913.
103 *Jewish Chronicle*, 21/11/1913.
104 Gerry Black, *op.cit.*, p.100.
105 *Jewish Chronicle*, 1/4/1921.

CHAPTER FOUR

Health and Hygiene

'The women of Glasgow might learn a good deal from Jewish mothers.'
Dr. Syme, Ruskin Society, Glasgow 1911

'It is fallacious to assert that the alien will eventually be the equal or the superior of the native population when the environment has had time to work its ameliorating effects.'
Karl Pearson and Margaret Moul, *Annals of Eugenics*, Vol.1, 1925–6, p.124

During the immigrant period the Jewish community had both supporters and detractors. Claims of insanitary habits were commonly made and were rebutted frequently. However, the allegation made in July 1910 that Jewish children in Glasgow were drinking methylated spirits had no basis in fact and was clearly anti-Semitic in intent.[1] Based on eugenics studies, Dr. David Heron carried out work in 1910 on the influence of 'defective physique and unfavourable home environment on the intelligence of schoolchildren'. He concluded, as would Pearson and Moul writing a decade later, that intelligence was hereditary and racial and that Jewish immigrant children compared unfavourably with Scottish children from Aberdeen, Edinburgh and Glasgow.[2] However, there were real concerns about the health of British children in the first years of the twentieth century after a relatively high number of potential recruits failed the fitness test for entry to the army during the Boer War of 1899–1902. The evidence as presented to the Report of the Interdepartmental Committee on Physical Deterioration in 1904 clearly indicated that Jewish children, all over Britain, were better fed than non-Jewish children.[3] We will see in more detail in Chapter 5 how the eugenists' attitudes to Jewish eyes and eye disease influenced the debate on health and alien immigration.

A more sympathetic view was that expressed by Dr. Syme of the Ruskin Society who referred, at a meeting in Glasgow in January 1911, to there being

> something interesting and mysterious about the Jew. English-born (sic) Jews were cleanly in their habits but the Continental Jews, or at least those with whom, in his hospital work he had come in contact were not so . . . there was no Jewish racial immunity from certain infectious diseases . . . superiority was due to the greater care taken by Jewish mothers of their children, especially in diet, and to the activities of the many Jewish associations and societies. The women of Glasgow might learn a good deal from Jewish mothers.[4]

The relative good health of the Jewish immigrants, despite living in poverty with insanitary habits, was a puzzle to many observers and it was usually attributed to better diet and personal hygiene.[5] Details of comparative statistics of aspects of Jewish health in Glasgow for this period are scanty but there were indications, made at the time, that infant mortality was lower within the Jewish community possibly by as much as one third.[6] In his evidence to the Interdepartmental Committee on Physical Deterioration, Dr. A. K. Chalmers, Medical Officer of Health for Glasgow, put the better health and nutritional status of the children of Jewish immigrants down to the fact that '. . . the immigrant is vigorous with a definite intention of bettering himself. That is why he comes here'.[7]

During the first years of the twentieth century figures kept by the Glasgow United Synagogue showed that births averaged 290 per year, giving a birth rate of 41 per thousand, given a Jewish community of about 7,000. These figures are broadly comparable to London Jewish birthrates[8] but considerably higher than that in the general Glasgow population. The Glasgow birth rate, 35.5 per thousand in 1876, had fallen to 25.5 by 1914. The Jewish death rate for the period was around 12 per thousand with a substantial proportion of the deaths, at least two thirds, in children under the age of 16. These figures confirm the youthful nature of the immigrant generation, mainly young adults with many children and accompanied by very few elderly relatives.

During the first years of the twentieth century, 1900 and 1901, the Jewish infant mortality rate, that is for stillbirths and children under the age of one year, was about 90 per thousand live births.[9] These rates were broadly similar to those of about twenty years earlier, at about 92 per thousand live births, when the Jewish community was far smaller. These figures confirm the contemporary impressions of Jewish death rates lower by one third, as the appalling Scottish infant mortality figures indicate that 13% of children (130 per thousand) died before their first birthday in 1895–1899, with the figures little changed over the next five years.[10] These figures have been blamed on Glasgow's poor and overcrowded housing stock which left a bitter legacy in terms of mortality and morbidity. The Jewish figures show that Jewish births and child mortality in Glasgow, despite the conditions experienced by the newcomers, mirrored developments around the Jewish immigrant world.

In examining figures for Jews and non-Jews in London and Manchester and in selected cities with a substantial Jewish population, such as Budapest, Amsterdam and eight American cities, Lara Marks related the lower Jewish infant mortality rates to behavioural, rather than environmental, factors.[11] She did not find that overcrowding put Jewish infants at a disadvantage but considered that the inspections of the Jewish Board of Guardians, which could lead to real improvements for the families visited, were of major importance. Religious factors may also have been important such as ritual hand washing before meals. Children may also have been protected by a longer period of maternal breastfeeding.[12] In Leeds it was discovered that Jewish rates of rickets were extremely low and that this might explain their lower risk of death from infectious disease.[13] In Glasgow too it was noted, in a study of children admitted to Belvedere Hospital, that the Jewish rate for rickets was substantially below that of the general population.[14] We have seen too that lower numbers of Jewish women in Glasgow were working outside the home and that even in cramped Gorbals conditions there were young Scottish or Irish girls living in to help with the family.

Studies in Glasgow had long shown the poor physique of working-class children. Many measures, including exercise, were proposed as possible remedies but Glasgow's health only began to improve in 1906–7 with such measures as the Schools' Medical Services and free school meals and milk which confronted the main problem, that of poverty, head on.[15] The Glasgow Jewish community shared concerns about the need for health improvement, and its solutions often paralleled developments in the general community. Dorothy Lindsay's studies of Jewish diet had indicated that Jews were better fed with a more balanced diet than their Gorbals neighbours but it was clear that additional factors could also be important.

The Glasgow Jewish Lads' Brigade, founded in May 1903, modelled itself on the Boys' Brigade and had the dual responsibility of providing discipline, citizenship and loyalty while aiding the acculturation of the immigrant young. The Brigade quickly became popular with Jewish boys in the Gorbals though often with an adult leadership drawn from Garnethill. While its aim of developing loyal Britons was openly stated, the benefit of producing fitter, and thus healthier, young men was also obvious. A non-Jewish officer, Lieutenant-Colonel I. H. Galbraith, visiting the Glasgow JLB in July 1919, commented that it was '. . . such a fine company . . . I hope that parents will realise what a splendid opportunity their sons are having of getting not only their bodies but their minds moulded and disciplined through the training received'.[16]

The sponsorship of athletic and other sporting activities by Jewish community organisations was often referred to as 'muscular Judaism'. Programmes of exercise for puny slum dwellers were often derided as an irrelevance.[17] However, a key Jewish objective was promoting fitness and health, while keeping young Jews within the framework of the community. Indeed, the early Glasgow Zionist movement believed that their support of the official Zionist political programme had to be supplemented by moves designed to improve the physical lot of the Jewish masses. Thus youngsters were encouraged to involve themselves in physical activity, and a Glasgow Zionist Cycling and Athletic Club was established in March 1899 with its own distinctive Zionist badge and uniform.[18]

If exercise was one health solution for the weak and undernourished, the idea of providing an annual holiday for slum children in the countryside also had its proponents. Some, however, rejected the idea as a distraction from the real need to provide permanent improvements in housing and nutrition.[19] Nevertheless, it would have seemed prudent for most mothers to permit their children to accept whatever benefits were available despite the suggestion of tokenism. In August 1908 fifty-seven poor Jewish children were taken for a two-week holiday in the country by the newly formed Glasgow Jewish Children's Fresh Air Fund. They were accommodated in a home rented from the missionary organisation, the Glasgow United Evangelical Association in West Kilbride, where 'every facility was offered for the observance of the Jewish dietary laws'.[20] This provision was important as the Fund had been set up to meet the religious needs of Jewish children from the Gorbals who had previously been sent to homes which were not under Jewish religious supervision. Supported from 1919 by the Boot and Clothing Fund of the Glasgow Jewish Board of Guardians, and the Glasgow Corporation, the 'fresh air' holidays remained popular and continued in the same format until the Second World War.[21]

Jewish children could be at risk in other ways too. They might be sent out on errands to help their parents, especially those involved in peddling. Manny Shinwell recalled travelling as a boy of 12 to California, a small village near Falkirk, to deliver goods for his father and to collect payment.[22] The sending of children on distant errands was not without its dangers, and one young Jewish girl, also aged 12, was murdered in Whiteinch in 1922 for the £2 she had just collected.[23]

Infectious Diseases

Britain's measures to deal with cholera, and other serious imported diseases, improved during the nineteenth century, moving from crude quarantine arrangements to more specific measures.[24] The great outbreak in London in 1866 affected the Jewish community there, and we shall see how the Jewish Glasgow-born physician, Dr. Asher Asher, and the London Jewish Board of Guardians took effective measures to deal with that situation. The public health infrastructure was improving all the time and, despite frequent subsequent cholera epidemics in Eastern Europe, Britain was to remain relatively free of the condition. The key lessons of the 1866 cholera epidemic centred on the provision of a clean, safe public water supply and the regulation of shipping into British ports.[25]

The Public Health Act of 1875 provided for the compulsory hospitalisation of travellers on ships with infectious diseases. The port authorities were given the powers to notify and isolate infectious cases.[26] The regulations, however, had to be strengthened in 1885, giving authorities greater compulsory rights to deal with infected travellers, including removal to hospital, provision of free medication and dealing with infected articles. In about 1870 the Medical Officer of Health for Glasgow, Dr. James Russell, recorded that relapsing fever had been brought to London by Polish Jewish immigrants, a claim rejected by the London Jewish Board of Guardians.[27] From London it arrived in Glasgow, infecting a large number of people. There remained concern about the number of travellers from Russia passing through Glasgow in the 1890s on account of the prevalence of serious infections such as cholera and typhus, and a special sanitary inspector was appointed to keep a watch on the lodging houses where the transmigrants stayed. Indeed, the only cholera cases diagnosed in Glasgow after 1866 were in two Jewish transmigrants, who had contracted the disease in Altona near Hamburg, during their travels on their way to America in August 1892.[28] The final great European pandemic of cholera had begun in the spring of 1892 and Hamburg was particularly affected, with almost 17,000 cases and a 50% mortality.[29] Britain, being on the transmigration route to North America, was particularly vulnerable, but the low incidence of cases in Britain and Glasgow's experience of only two cases, was fairly typical. It showed that the disease could be isolated despite its prevalence in Europe. Further measures of control in subsequent years confirmed the ability of the public health authorities to identify and control the problem. By 1896 Russia was declared free of cholera and the public fears of the regular return of cholera from the transmigrants was finally allayed.

It was perhaps surprising that there had not been more cases. Conditions on the ships crossing the North Sea to Scotland were just as cramped and insanitary as on those sailing the Atlantic. We have already seen that passengers arriving at Leith in 1891 were weakened by the crossing and some had to be hospitalised. Steerage accommodation consisted of dormitories close to benches and tables set aside for meals. Food was basic: herring, potatoes and black bread. For the ten-day-long trans-Atlantic crossing Jewish passengers, avoiding non-kosher food, troubled by seasickness and existing in insanitary conditions, would have eaten little, further contributing to their weakened state.

With the Infectious Disease (Notification) Act, originally passed in 1889 and made obligatory by resolution of Glasgow Corporation in 1890, it was possible to monitor the course of infection. Previously it had been necessary to wait to use registers of deaths to identify illness although it was recognised that falling death rates did not always correlate with a falling prevalence of illness.[30] The regulations were flexible enough to permit additional diseases to be added as required and cholera was added temporarily during 1892 when the two cases already referred to were diagnosed. Later such conditions as pulmonary tuberculosis (1910) and trachoma (1914) were added. This gave the Glasgow authorities powers to deal with conditions for which there had previously been no hospital provision, unless the patient qualified for poor-law medical relief or could obtain admission to a general hospital.

In America the arrival of ships containing immigrants in 1892 carrying typhus and cholera led to President Harrison halting immigration temporarily, and quarantine measures were instituted. It was tacitly accepted that the steerage immigrants were the disease vector needing to be quarantined, although there was little scientific bacteriological evidence to support the assumption.[31] Local and national health authorities specifically targeted immigrant Jews from Eastern Europe, though they were only about 10% of all immigrants to the United States in 1892. Jews were removed both from incoming ships and from their new homes in New York. Those rounded up were sent to nearby designated quarantine islands, and the quarantine regulations reduced the flow of immigrants to America to a trickle.[32] Eventually the Americans passed a National Quarantine Act. The legislation specified regulation and disinfection, rather than immigration restriction, and provided proper protocols for inspection and sanitation with an immigration halt as a final sanction.

Typhus, a louse-borne rickettsial infection, owed much in its endemic form in Britain to conditions in the individual industrial cities with occasional escalation during periods of disruption. Despite the crowded conditions in areas of the major cities, including the Gorbals in Glasgow where the immigrant Jews settled, typhus steadily disappeared after 1880. This can be credited to the vigilance of the health authorities and also indicates that Jewish immigrants were not a major cause of social and economic dislocation in which typhus could have been expected to flourish.[33] Typhoid was a major problem in Jewish immigrant areas, with the influx aggravating existing sanitary problems as the supposed relative Jewish immunity to cholera and typhus did not extend to typhoid.[34] Nevertheless, Hardy concludes that the major Jewish immigration to London of the 1890s had a minimal epidemiological and demographic impact,[35] and the Glasgow experience is not likely to have been any different.

Despite additional sanitary inspection, more serious epidemics continued to affect Glasgow. The most serious was the reappearance of plague in the city in August and September 1900, thought to have been caused by infected rats from a cargo ship from Oporto in Portugal.[36] Though the centre of the outbreak occurred in Rose

Street and Thistle Street in the Gorbals, in the heart of the local Jewish community, there were no Jewish patients.[37] Venereal diseases were also reckoned to be low in the Jewish community. In New York it was noted that the social dislocations of immigration had caused an increase in such diseases in the Jewish population but levels were still low when compared to other groups.[38] Provision was made for local treatment for steerage passengers at the Glasgow docks but really the major port incidence was rather in the seamen than in the passengers. Thus a memorandum in November 1918 indicated that 'so far, the occurrence of venereal disease in immigrants has not come prominently before this department'.[39]

Tuberculosis

Despite a major improvement in tuberculosis mortality in Glasgow in the last decades of the nineteenth century, tuberculosis remained a major killer, still responsible for 13% of all deaths in Scotland in the 1890s.[40] By this time cholera had disappeared from Glasgow and typhus had all but been eradicated.[41] The incidence of tuberculosis was also decreasing in Glasgow but, given its previous high level there, it had further to fall than in most other centres. Thus the main period of Jewish growth in Glasgow coincided with a substantial drop in infectious disease.

It might be expected that the first generation of Jewish immigrants to Glasgow, crowded into Gorbals tenements and employed in sweated tailoring workshops, might have had a high incidence of mortality from tuberculosis. However, studies carried out in the first years of the twentieth century in many diverse areas of major urban Jewish concentrations around the world showed that mortality from tuberculosis among Jews was only a half, and in cities like Krakow and even Vienna, only about a third that of their non-Jewish neighbours. In London, the Jewish rate was about a quarter less than that of non-Jews, and United Synagogue burial returns a decade before, in the early 1890s, showed a Jewish mortality from tuberculosis only half that for the general populations.[42] While no statistics of Jews with tuberculosis are available for Glasgow, this impression of low mortality was recognised in 1917 by Roderick Scott, Convener of the Glasgow Public Health Committee.[43]

Glasgow itself, through its municipal government and powerful public health movement, played a leading role in the anti-tuberculosis crusade of the 1890s. Koch's discovery of the tubercle bacillus in 1882, proving that the disease was infectious and did not have a hereditary basis, came as no surprise to Dr. James Russell, Glasgow Medical Officer of Health. Russell had noted early on the link between the disease and overcrowding and was involved in sanitary and public health measures to reduce mortality.[44] However, it was clear in any of the Jewish immigrant areas in Britain that there was a significant morbidity from tuberculosis. Indeed, it was assumed that the disease ran a more chronic course in Jewish patients. Feldman's own enquiries at the Whitechapel Tuberculosis Dispensary confirmed the number of Jewish tuberculosis patients whose disease ran for many years without the sufferer being unduly incapacitated.[45] Feldman examined a number of theories for the low Jewish mortality, and after some fanciful ones had been eliminated he indicated his belief that ultimately the Jews benefited from sobriety, good maternal care and a low incidence of syphilis. Similar low levels of Jewish TB deaths had also been identified in the United States where economic and hygienic factors were also adduced.[46] Another theory advanced was the long Jewish exposure to urban life, and thus also to the disease.[47]

By the first years of the twentieth century better facilities existed for the care of Jewish tuberculosis sufferers. In London the Jewish Board of Guardians visited homes to advise on health measures, such as the reduction of overcrowding and promotion of hygiene. Patients could be sent to sanatoria or boarded out in the country although about as many were sent to hospitals and infirmaries. While the London Board was not usually noted for its proactive approach to health problems, the combination of a Jewish health problem and the lack of statutory provision provoked them into action. In Glasgow too the Board of Guardians was the leading

Jewish agency in the fight against tuberculosis. As Dr. Syme had pointed out, a key factor in better Jewish health was the supportive role of the Jewish agencies. They sponsored home treatment measures that formed a major part of local expenditure on tuberculosis sufferers with regular weekly and monthly grants and the direct provision of additional food. Measures to reduce the heavy ongoing expenditure were regularly considered to try to ease the considerable strain on the Board's resources.[48] One promising suggestion was to send consumptives on to parts of the Empire where the climate might help to effect a cure, and a number of people were assisted to settle in Australia or the Orange Free State.[49] There are no figures to give an indication of the numbers of Jewish consumptives in Glasgow although there was enough of a problem for the Board of Guardians to designate their ambitious Special Jubilee Fund in 1916 for tuberculosis relief and the following year to set up a Consumption Committee.

The Special Jubilee Fund was designed to raise enough money, estimated to be about £3,000, to enable local consumptives to settle in warmer climates. There was a long history in Britain of promoting emigration, especially to Australia and New Zealand, as a climatic cure for tuberculosis although there were conflicting claims about the value of such migration, both for the patient and for the health of the destination society.[50] The Jewish Board of Guardians actually believed 1916 to be their golden jubilee year but in fact, as we have seen, the origins of the Board can be safely dated back to even before 1858. The problem of Jewish paupers with tuberculosis had become a major one by the First World War. Increasing numbers were requiring hospitalisation in Glasgow and their families required regular relief from the Jewish Board of Guardians. It was felt that the drain on the Jewish communal purse could only be eased by the encouragement of emigration, and although the fund did not reach the £3,000 target, £850 was quickly raised. It was estimated that it would cost between £70 and £100 to resettle a family abroad and support them until they could become independent, and so the Special Jubilee Fund should have helped to resettle about forty families.

It had been recognised in both Glasgow and London that merely paying for sanatorium care and medical treatment was not sufficient, as many with tuberculosis relapsed when returning home to work.[51] This movement of the Jewish consumptives out of Glasgow had long-term benefits for the health of the community. Within ten years of the end of the war city health statistics confirmed that Jews had a lower incidence of tuberculosis than their non-Jewish neighbours.[52] Glasgow's poor reputation for tuberculosis was earned especially during the interwar years, by which time Jewish sufferers, and the proportion of Glasgow's Jews in the most overcrowded parts of the Gorbals, were much less numerous. By 1930 there were only 22 cases (4.23%) of tuberculosis dealt with by the Glasgow Jewish Board of Guardians out of a total caseload of 521.[53]

By March 1917 about half of the target of £3,000 for the Special Jubilee Fund had been collected, although little headway was made in raising the outstanding balance even one year later.[54] Money from the 'Consumptive Fund' was used to send sufferers to sanatoria or to parts of the South of England where the climate was better than in Glasgow. About twenty Jewish patients from Glasgow with tuberculosis were being supported financially in sanatoria in 1917.[55] However, the Glasgow Jewish Board of Guardians Report for 1918 expressed the hope that the end of wartime travelling restrictions, and the raising of further funds, would mean that patients could be helped emigrate. The general demands on the Board continued to increase at a rapid rate and the burden of tuberculosis relief remained heavy. Louis Abrahams, Honorary Treasurer of the Glasgow Board, commented that 'the Board does not receive all it should and it could spend very much more than it gets but the present progress tends in the right direction'.[56]

The Poorhouse and Poor Relief

The spirit of Scottish poor relief was rooted in values shared by Jews as well as Scots, namely thrift and self-help with the support and encouragement of the religious authorities, whether of the synagogue or of the kirk. With increasing urbanisation in the nineteenth century the old Scottish voluntary structures gave way after 1845 to a system providing medical relief for the sick poor.[57] The poor, but only the poor, now had free access to parochial medical services as well as to hospitals, including asylums for mental illness. In Scotland the poor looked for aid to the community where they were known and where care specific to their needs could be given.[58] This too matched the Jewish welfare system, based as it was on a defined community supported by local, though often limited, resources.

It was Govan Parish, covering the Gorbals as well as Govan and Partick, which was responsible for the area which included the majority of the immigrant Jewish community. The most important facility provided by the Parish was the outdoor medical service, which was preferred by the poor to indoor relief as it, preserved their dignity by enabling them to remain in the community.[59] While the Jewish newcomers found an available system of parochial care, from 1889, under the control of parish councils, they did not find one which always provided a high standard of service.

The Jews, or their supporters, sometimes claimed that no Jews were obtaining Poor Relief. It was certainly true that only small numbers availed themselves of this provision, preferring instead to use Jewish agencies where available. Settlement laws meant that from 1845 there had to be three years' residence before paupers could claim relief, though this was reduced in 1898. Indeed, parishes could not help more than a small proportion of those who might need assistance, while admission to the hospital wards or a poorhouse carried a stigma.[60] In 1902, for example, alien Jews made up only 28 out of the 5,656 applicants for Poor Relief, just about half of one per cent, a proportion much less even than that of Jews in the Gorbals. Of these 28, three required care in the lunatic asylum while 18 received indoor relief.[61]

The numbers of Jews in care at the Merryflatts Hospital in Govan, which catered for 'pauper lunatics', that is those poor with psychiatric problems, the destitute and those with TB, increased slowly from the 1890s onwards, part of a general increase in the numbers seeking entry to the poorhouse. The total of Jewish admissions rarely exceeded thirty in a year with only one or two long-term inmates amongst them.[62] Given the number of immigrant Jews who could have formed a charge on the welfare facilities of the wider community, these figures confirm that the Jewish uptake of Poor Relief or admissions to Merryflatts was below their relative proportion in the city. The safety net provided by the Jewish Board of Guardians and the other Jewish welfare associations undoubtedly enabled many Jews to avoid parochial relief.

Hospitals

The Victoria Infirmary and Merryflatts Poorhouse, later the Southern General Hospital, dealt with the majority of hospitalised members of the community, based as they were on the southern side of the city. Visiting hours in hospital were strictly enforced at this time and relatives were not allowed to bring in food. Observant Jewish patients found many problems with hospital meals, both from the unfamiliarity with the Scottish diet as well as from the lack of *kashrut*. Besides the obvious difficulty with religious observance it was felt that eating gentile food would be a hindrance to convalescence.[63] Arrangements had been in existence in Manchester for many years for the provision of kosher food and for observance of Shabbat and the Festivals in the Bridge Street Workhouse.[64] The Jewish authorities in Manchester found it convenient to refer cases to the Workhouse, especially those who did not fit easily into the system operated by the Jewish Board of Guardians or who were simply troublemakers'.[65]

The moves for a kosher kitchen in Glasgow received help from James Weir, a surgeon at the Victoria Infirmary. Weir took an active interest in the welfare of his many Jewish patients and served as Medical Officer to the Jewish friendly societies that were affiliated to the parent body, the Order of Ancient Maccabeans. Unfortunately Weir migrated to Australia in April 1910 before any final decision was made.[66] However, when formally approached by

Rev. E.P. Phillips on behalf of the Jewish community for the provision of kosher food, the privately endowed Victoria Infirmary declined the request. They were unwilling to commit themselves to the provision of a service which they felt might lead to them having to offer additional facilities to the Jewish or other communities in the future. There was no complaint about Jewish treatment in the hospitals but many of the Jewish patients were brought up from childhood to observe the Jewish dietary laws strictly and the strange diet was felt to be a hindrance to recovery.[67]

In the end it was the Merryflatts Poorhouse, run by Glasgow Corporation, which agreed to permit the opening of a kosher kitchen, under the supervision of Rabbi Hillman, in January 1914.[68] This kitchen, achieved by patient negotiation conducted by Bernard Glasser with the hospital authorities and Dr. A. K. Chalmers, the Medical Officer of Health for Glasgow, was still functioning twenty-five years later. The Jewish Hospital Fund and Sick Visiting Association then requested the Victoria Infirmary to bring in kosher food to the hospital from outside, presumably from Merryflatts. A meeting of the Infirmaries Consultative Committee, which represented the Victoria, Western and Royal Infirmaries, took place in 1915 and '. . . after some discussion it was unanimously agreed not to entertain the application as there had been no difficulty in the past with Jewish patients taking the ordinary food'.[69]

There was little evidence of Jewish immigrants being especially prone to the infectious diseases afflicting Glasgow at the end of the nineteenth century and in the first decades of the twentieth century. Despite immigrant poverty and overcrowding, Jews were affected less by outbreaks of infectious disease and it was generally acknowledged, in a wide variety of urban centres, that Jews had a lower incidence of tuberculosis than the general population. However, there was one infectious disease, trachoma, uniquely visible, which campaigners against Jewish immigration must have felt gave their cause support, and this will be examined next.

TABLE 4.1 *Jewish Statistics in Glasgow, 1902–1904*

	Circumcisions	*marriages*	*deaths excl. stillbirths*
1902	166	76	85
1903	132	60	84
1904	147	36	88

Source: Minute Book of the United Synagogue of Glasgow, 1898–1906, SJAC

TABLE 4.2 *Records of Jewish Deaths in Glasgow*

	Still-born	*below 1 year*	*1 to 16 years*	*adult*	*total*
C, J 1884	2	4	7	7	20
C, J 1885	1	2	2	7	12
W, J 1900	4	15	15	14	48
W, J 1901	10	24	21	22	77
S 1908	4	28	13	14	59

Source: Records of deaths of Jewish cemeteries in Scotland, SJAC

C: Craigton, J: Janefield (Eastern Necropolis), W: Western Necropolis (Maryhill), S: Sandymount

TABLE 4.3 *Jewish Births in Glasgow*

1884: 38
1885: 27

Source: Births Register of the Glasgow Hebrew Congregation, SJAC

TABLE 4.4 *Steerage Passengers Arriving in New York in 1891*

Port of origin	*numbers*	*%*
Liverpool	110,000	27.3
Hamburg	82,000	20.3
Bremen	68,000	16.9
Rotterdam	25,000	6.2
Le Havre	25,000	6.2
Glasgow	23,000	5.7
Mediterranean ports	50,000	12.4
Other North European ports	20,000	5.0
Total	403,000	100.0

In 1891 over 560,000 immigrants arrived in the United States, 12.3% of whom were Jewish.

Source: Howard Markel, *Quarantine! East European Jewish Immigrants and the New York City Epidemics of 1892* (Baltimore, 1997), pp.141–142

References

1 *Jewish Chronicle*, 22/7/1910.
2 David Heron, 'The Influence of Defective Physique and Unfavourable Home Environment on the Intelligence of Schoolchildren', *Eugenics Laboratory Memoirs, VIII* (Cambridge, 1910), pp.58–59.
3 Interdepartmental Committee on Physical Deterioration, PP, 1904, Vol. XXXII, Part 2, Cd 2210. Most of those interviewed on the nutrition of Jewish children confirmed that they were better fed than non-Jewish children. Typical is the evidence of Mrs. Close (Q2772): 'The Jewish children are incomparably better fed - women have a strong sense of religious duty'.
4 *Jewish Chronicle*, 20/1/1911.
5 Anne Hardy, *The Epidemic Streets: Infectious Disease and the Rise of Preventive Medicine 1856–1900* (Oxford, 1993), p.287.
6 Rev. Louis Morris, address to Glasgow Jewish Literary Society, reported in *Jewish Chronicle*, 25/2/1916.
7 Report of the Interdepartmental Committee on Physical Deterioration, PP, 1904, Vol XXXII, Part 2, Cd 2210. Evidence of Dr. A K Chalmers (Q6090).
8 Lara Marks, *Model Mothers: Jewish Mothers and Maternity Provision in East London 1870–1939* (Oxford, 1994), p.84.
9 Jewish infant mortality data compiled from records of United Synagogue of Glasgow 1898–1906; Births, Marriages and Deaths Registers of the Glasgow Hebrew Congregation 1884–1885, Records of the Jewish Cemeteries of Scotland, at SJAC. With smaller numbers of births and deaths in the nineteenth century and some under-reporting of Garnethill records, early figures are less accurate.
10 David Hamilton, *The Healers: A History of Medicine in Scotland* (Edinburgh,1981), p.236.
11 Lara Marks, *op.cit.,* pp.64–65.
12 Report of the Interdepartmental Committee on Physical Deterioration, PP 1904, Vol XXXII, Part 2, Q452.
13 Marks, *op.cit.*, pp.73–74.
14 Alexander Macgregor, 'Physique of Glasgow Children admitted to the City of Glasgow Fever Hospital, Belvedere during the years 1907–1908', *Royal Philosophical Society of Glasgow*, Vol.40, 1908, p.172.
15 David Hamilton, *op.cit.*, p.241.
16 *Jewish Chronicle*, 29/3/1918.
17 David Hamilton, *op.cit.*, p.241.
18 Kenneth Collins, *Second City Jewry: the Jews of Glasgow in the Age of Expansion 1790–1919* (Glasgow, 1990), p.118.
19 Ralph Glasser, *Growing up in the Gorbals* (London, 1986), pp.54–55.
20 *Jewish Chronicle*, 7/8/1908.
21 *Jewish Chronicle*, 25/7/1919; Kenneth Collins, 'The Growth and Development of Scottish Jewry', in Kenneth Collins ed., *Aspects of Scottish Jewry* (Glasgow, 1987), p.34.
22 Emmanuel Shinwell, *Conflict Without Malice* (London, 1955), p.21.
23 M Anne Crowther and Brenda White, *On Soul and Conscience: the Medical Expert and Crime* (Aberdeen, 1988), p.56.

24 J C McDonald, 'The History of Quarantine in Britain during the 19th Century', *Bulletin of the History of Medicine*, Vol.25, 1951, pp.22–44.
25 Anne Hardy, 'Cholera, quarantine and the English preventive system 1850–1895', *Medical History*, Vol.37, 1993, pp.250–269.
26 Anne Hardy, *op.cit.*, p.258.
27 Edna Roberston, *Glasgow's Doctor: James Burn Russell* (East Linton, 1998), p.149. LJBG Medical Committee refutation of rumour of relapsing fever in Jewish immigrants from Poland, in Mordechai Rozin, *The Rich and the Poor: Jewish Philanthropy and Social Control in Nineteenth-Century London* (Brighton,1999), p.179.
28 A K Chalmers, ed., *Public Health Administration in Glasgow: A Memorial Volume of the Writings of James Burn Russell* (Glasgow, 1905), p.358.
29 Anne Hardy, *op.cit.*, pp.261–262.
30 A.K Chalmers, *The Health of Glasgow: 1818–1925, An Outline* (Glasgow, 1930), pp.292–295.
31 Howard Markel, *Quarantine! East European Jewish Immigrants and the New York City Epidemics of 1892* (Baltimore, 1997) p.122.
32 *Ibid.*, p.134.
33 Anne Hardy, 'Urban famine or urban crisis? Typhus in the Victorian city', in R J Morris and Richard Rodger (eds.) *The Victorian City: A Reader in British Urban History 1820–1914* (London,1993), p.240.
34 Anne Hardy, *Epidemic Streets*, pp.178–181.
35 Anne Hardy, *ibid.*, p.287.
36 Alexander Macgregor, *Public Health in Glasgow: 1905–1946* (Edinburgh,1967), p.6.
37 Royal Commission on Alien Immigration, 1903, evidence of Julius Pinto, 20871–20874.
38 Deborah Dwork, 'Health Conditions of Immigrant Jews on the Lower East Side of New York: 1880–1914', *Medical History*, 1981, Vol.25, p.31.
39 A K Chalmers, *op.cit.*, p.391.
40 David Hamilton, *op.cit.*, p.236.
41 Edna Robertson, *op.cit.*, p.149.
42 W M Feldman, 'Tuberculosis and the Jew', in *The Tuberculosis Year Book*, Vol.1, 1913–1914, pp.48–54; Anne Hardy, *Epidemic Streets*, p.289.
43 *Jewish Chronicle*, 14/9/1917.
44 Edna Robertson, *op.cit.*, pp.144–149.
45 W M Feldman, *op.cit.*, pp.48–54.
46 Michael E Teller, *The Tuberculosis Movement: A Public Health Campaign in the Progressive Era* (New York,1988), p.98; Theodore B Sachs, 'Tuberculosis in the Jewish District of Chicago', *JAMA*, 1904, Vol.43, p.390.
47 Teller, *op.cit.*, p.97; Lilian Brandt, *The Social Aspects of Tuberculosis: based on a study of statistics*, Committee on Tuberculosis, 1902, pp.31–115.
48 Glasgow Jewish Board of Guardians, Annual Reports, 1912–1916.
49 *Ibid*; *Jewish Chronicle*, 29/9/1916.
50 Linda Bryder, '"A Health Resort for Consumptives": Tuberculosis and Immigration to New Zealand, 1880–1914', *Medical History*, 1996, Vol.40, pp.453–471.
51 *Jewish Chronicle*, 29/9/1916.
52 *Jewish Echo*, 28/11/1930.

53 *Jewish Chronicle*, 16/3/1917.
54 *Jewish Chronicle*, 25/5/1917.
55 Kenneth Collins, *Second City Jewry*, *op.cit.*, p.196.
56 Stephanie Blackden, 'The Poor Law and Health: A Survey of Parochial Medical Aid in Glasgow, 1845–1900', in T C Smout, (ed.), *The Search for Wealth and Stability, Essays in Economic and Social History presented to M W Flinn* (London, 1979), p.243.
57 M Anne Crowther, 'Poverty, Health and Welfare', in W Hamish Fraser and R J Morris, (eds.), *People and Society in Scotland, Volume II, 1830–1914* (Edinburgh, 1990), p.273.
58 Stephanie Blackden, *op.cit.*, p.249.
59 *Ibid*, p.262.
60 *Glasgow Municipal Commission on Housing for the Poor* (Glasgow, 1904), pp.220, 232.
61 Records of the Merryflatts Combination Poorhouse 1886–1914, GGHB Archives, Mitchell Library.
62 *Jewish Chronicle*, 9/9/1910.
63 Rainer Liedtke, *Jewish Welfare in Hamburg and Manchester c1850–1914* (Oxford, 1998), p.104.
64 Rainer Liedtke, *op.cit.*, p.107.
65 *Jewish Chronicle*, 8/4/1910.
66 *British Medical Journal*, 24/9/1910, 1910, Vol.2, p.901.
67 *Jewish Chronicle*, 16/1/1914.
68 'Bernard Glasser at 85', *Jewish Echo*, 20/9/1957.
69 (Glasgow) Infirmaries Consultative Committee, in Glasgow Royal Infirmary Minutes, 17/11/1915, GGHB Archives, Mitchell Library.

CHAPTER FIVE

Trachoma

'The time comes to go on board the ship. People tell them that they should take a walk to the doctor. So they go to the doctor. The doctor examines them and finds that they are all hale and hearty and can go to America but she, that is Goldele, cannot go because she has trachomas on her eyes. At first her family do not understand. Only later do they realise it. That meant that they could all go to America, but she, Goldele, would have to remain here in Antwerp. So there began a wailing, a weeping, a moaning. Three times her mama fainted. Her papa wanted to stay here, but he couldn't. All the ship tickets would be lost. So they had to go off to America and leave her, Goldele, here until the trachomas would go away from her eyes.'

Sholom Aleichem, 'Off for the Golden Land', *Jewish Immigration Bulletin*, February 1917, p.10

'. . . how far the poor sight of the Jews reaches back to their oriental racial origins or is a product of centuries of ghetto life is impossible to predict . . . our data seem to indicate that poor eyesight is not the product of the immediate environment . . . rather a racial character modified by selective action throughout many generations . . .'

Karl Pearson and Margaret Maul, *Annals of Eugenics*, Volume 3, 1928, p.254

Trachoma in Glasgow around the turn of the twentieth century linked three distinct geographical areas: Eastern Europe, a reservoir of patients, many of whose inhabitants were on the move westwards; the United States, destination for so many European immigrants, which was becoming increasingly concerned about the health of its citizens; and Glasgow, on one of the transmigrant routes, and temporary home to thousands of aliens, some harbouring infection, who intended at some stage to complete their journey by crossing the Atlantic. Indeed, it was the belief that there was a substantial number of alien Jews suffering from trachoma that brought the disease to the fore during the debate on the Aliens Bill as it passed through Parliament during 1905.

We have already seen that from the 1890s public and political clamour grew for restriction on the number of aliens allowed to enter Britain as Jewish immigration to Britain increased. The Scottish transmigrant route became established during the 1890s as Scottish shipping companies, like the Anchor and Allan lines, entered the transatlantic market. These lines competed for passengers with English companies, transporting migrants from Hull or London to Liverpool, before crossing the Atlantic, or Continental companies sailing direct from Hamburg, Rotterdam or Libau. We have also seen that the arguments for control of the Jewish influx were economic and social as well as medical, and the limited but definite presence of trachoma amongst the Jewish immigrants was given as one factor in the need for restriction of alien entry to Britain.[1]

Because of its peculiar visibility as a disease of the Jewish alien, trachoma was particularly attractive to those who saw medical grounds for excluding Jewish immigration as a more honourable cause than basing restrictions purely on racial grounds. Further, by pointing out the dangerous, infectious nature of the alien Jew with his contagious eye disease, it was possible to stoke the fires of contemporary anti-Semitism without seeming to deviate from the path of an accurate assessment of medical immigration statistics.

Jewish Eyes

Establishing medical criteria as the main grounds for permitting immigration had the advantage of removing the racial element from the discussion about limiting the numbers of newcomers to Britain. At the end of the nineteenth century and into the twentieth century various theories of psychobiological decline came together in the person of Francis Galton (1822–1911), a cousin of Charles Darwin.[2] A theory of eugenics developed which taught that survival lay in selective breeding. Racial origins mattered more to Galton as a cause of disease than the poor housing, sanitation and environment which medical officers of health like Dr. James Russell were working so hard to improve. The eugenists attempted to use their theories of racial purity in an attempt to keep what they considered to be the 'degenerate' alien Jews out of Britain. It seemed possible that in trachoma they might have a medical cause.

Writing in the *Annals of Eugenics* in the 1920s, but based on research carried out a decade earlier, Pearson and Moul looked at whether an already crowded country like Britain could permit 'indiscriminate' immigration. They sought to identify grounds, 'without prejudice', using 'purely detached science', on which a discriminatory entry policy could be based.[3] They believed that Jews, as immigrants, were never absorbed, and remained a nation within a nation. Even worse, they feared that Jews might intermarry and create 'hybrids on which science could contribute little'. Pearson and Moul carried out large numbers of tests, including a detailed assessment of eyesight and other aspects of function of the eyes, on hundreds of Jewish schoolchildren in London. These tests, painstaking and tediously detailed, provoked fright, and occasionally even hysteria, during some of the eye testing, particularly when examining Jewish schoolgirls. Pearson and Moul concluded that their comparison of Jewish children with non-Jewish children from London and Leeds in England and from Aberdeen, Edinburgh and Glasgow showed that 'there can be no doubt of the superiority in eye healthiness of the average Gentile over the alien Jew'[4] and that 'our data seem to indicate that poor eyesight is not the product of the immediate environment . . . rather a racial character modified by selective action throughout many generations . . .'[5]

Jewish eyes were not just the subject of academic research. Indeed, the physiognomy of the Jew was also becoming a subject for study, both scientific and scurrilous, during the last years of the nineteenth century. The sight of the Jew could be seen as a truer indication of the Jews' real nature than any other obvious feature. Francis Galton tried to capture this Jewish appearance by making composite photographs of boys at the Jews' Free School in London in 1891.[6] In these pictures he thought he could see what he called the 'cold, scanning gaze' of the Jew as the sign of their difference, of their potential pathology. Thus, for Galton and his followers, Jewish eyes, or the Jewish gaze, did not just mark Jews out as looking identifiably, and ethnically, Jewish but also indicated that they also looked somehow 'inferior'.

Jewish social scientists of the period were also affected by Galton's finding of the 'Jewishness' of the gaze of Jewish eyes. Joseph Jacobs (1854–1916) was the first of the Jewish racial scientists to challenge the view that Jews were physically and mentally degenerate.[7] Rejecting the view of racial anti-Semites, Jacobs became an outspoken Jewish defender affording his people comfort and support. In 1891 Jacobs wrote that he failed to see 'any of the cold calculation which Mr. Galton noticed in the boys at the school' while acknowledging that in Galton's composite photographs 'those are Jewish eyes'.[8] Jacobs, as a contributor on Anthropological Types in the *Jewish Encyclopaedia* described Jewish eyes as

> . . . generally brilliant, both eyelids are heavy and bulging, and it seems to be the main characteristic of the Jewish eye that the upper lid covers a larger proportion of the pupil than among other persons. This may serve to give a sort of nervous, furtive look to the eyes, which, when the pupils are small and set close together with semistrabismus, gives keenness to some Jewish eyes.[9]

Gilman in referring to the images of Jewish eyes notes the positive, such as in Freud's dream of Herzl's 'infinitely sad eyes' and the idealised Jewish images of Ephraim Moses Lilien in *fin-de-siècle* Vienna, which aimed to counter the image of the Jew as diseased. The negative side, the 'melancholy, pained expression', appeared in the writings of such Jewish physicians as Moses Julius Gutman.[10] Thus, in the polemic language of the time, the Jew could not have a neutral gaze. The 'cold, scanning gaze', derided by the eugenist as pathological, was to form the structure of psychoanalysis. Some writers could see in the vivacity of the Jewish eye a sign of the remarkable Jewish persistence of hope in adversity, illustrated by the *Jewish Chronicle* description of Jewish and non-Jewish emigrants from Russia passing through Berlin in 1891. This contrasted the 'almost too intelligent Jewish eyes' with the vacant 'stare' of the gentile travellers.[11] Writers like Francis Galton could see only the pathology of the Jewish soul.

Trachoma in the United States

In 1891 United States law brought immigration under federal control and defined 'contagious disease' as grounds for refusing entry. Disease identification was removed from lay observers and placed in the hands of physicians who had jurisdiction over visible illness.[12] Immigrants refused entry in New York soon found their way back to Glasgow. In 1893, a case at the Glasgow Sheriff Court, Wallace v J. & A. Allan, established that shipping companies were under no legal obligation to return aliens from America to their country of origin, although they may have had a contractual obligation, under penalty from the Government, to do so.[13] Over the next twenty years the numbers rejected after medical inspections in the States rose from 0.77% in 1898 to 1.26% in 1909 and 2.78% in 1912.[14] Those refused entry were increasingly being excluded on medical grounds.

It was in 1898 that trachoma was recognised as a dangerous contagious disease in America. As an illness of the immigrant community, trachoma was highly visible and thus attracted fear as well as easy recognition, as victims carried the signs of the disease on the most prominent part of their faces - their eyes. Very quickly, the newly arrived Jewish immigrant personified the threat of trachoma for most Americans of the immigrant generation, and it was not just the native Americans who made this link.[15] The real risk of trachoma was well known to the Jewish immigrants and was well recognised in Scotland also. In 1900, more than a hundred Jewish emigrants from Britain were debarred from the United States on medical grounds.[16]

The incidence of trachoma and its potential to prevent Jews from Eastern Europe from being allowed to travel across Europe and to settle in the United States was well known thanks to a campaign of posters, publications and other information easily available in Russia. One popular booklet, *What Every Immigrant Should Know,* was widely distributed through the Jewish Pale of Settlement in Russia under the auspices of the American National Council of Jewish Women. This exhorted Jews with eye problems to think hard and to reconsider their plans for travel to the United States.[17] In 1898, the year that trachoma was recognised as a dangerous contagious disease in America, medical deportations from Ellis Island numbered 258, compared to only one the year before.[18] By 1903, the *Handbook of the Medical Examination of Immigrants* indicated that the purpose of the screening process was not only to prevent the introduction of communicable disease but 'also to keep out a class of people from whom so large a proportion of the inmates of institutions for the blind and recipients of public dispensary charity are recruited'.[19]

As Yew makes clear, the emphasis on the detection of trachoma on Ellis Island indicated the ascendancy of medicine through a shift in American public health policy towards immigrants. The eye inspection at Ellis Island was most feared, especially by Jews who formed a substantial majority of those detained by the physician:

> By a quick movement and the force of his own compelling gaze, he catches the eyes of his subject and holds them. You will see the immigrant stop short, lift his head with a quick jerk, and open his eyes very wide. The inspector reaches with a swift movement, catches the eyelash with his thumb and finger, turns it back and peers under it. If all is well the immigrant is passed on . . .[20]

From 1898 these medical inspections were carried out on the eyes of anyone with signs of corneal roughness or opacity, thickened or drooping lids or conjunctival congestion.[21] By 1905 all immigrants had to have their eyelids everted. Naturally, the numbers of medical officers required to process the continual flow of immigrants increased also. Despite the strict inspection procedures at Ellis Island trachoma was widespread in the immigrant population of the east-coast American cities. In 1905 a careful study of New York schoolchildren revealed that 4.2% had severe trachoma while 5.8% had mild trachoma.[22] Treacher Collins blamed much of this, however, on Irish rather than Jewish incomers, a source also of importance in Glasgow.[23] Indeed, in 1895 the incidence of trachoma in Ireland was three times that in Scotland.[24]

Shipping companies gradually increased their vigilance, trying to ensure that travellers were free of such illnesses as smallpox and typhoid, as well as trachoma, understanding that those who failed immigration medicals in America would be returned to their last European port of call at the company's expense. In practice this was hard to enforce. Many migrants travelled round many British and European ports prior to crossing the Atlantic, and defining the precise port of origin could be difficult. Thus, there was an increasing risk that immigrants with trachoma could accumulate in Britain at the expense of Poor Law bodies and Jewish Boards of Guardians around the country who might even find that they were left with the responsibility for the return journey across the Atlantic.[25]

Thus diseases like trachoma, carried by a number of transmigrants, only reached the attention of the authorities around the turn of the century. With large population groups on the move infection might easily reach a significant number of people before detection. It was reported in 1900 that no fewer than 330 would-be emigrants were turned back from the Russian border railway station at Thorn. The ability of the shipping companies to police infection control measures effectively was reduced by the *shleppern,* professional agents usually based in the larger towns along the major migration routes, helping would-be emigrants evade immigration inspection procedures.[26] However, in their enthusiasm to prevent the admission of trachoma sufferers shipping companies were often unwilling to take any risks at all. Thus those even with the most minor eye conditions, quite distinct from trachoma, were often prevented from travelling.[27]

Trachoma

Known widely as granular ophthalmia during the latter part of the nineteenth century, trachoma is an eye disease characterised by watering of the eyes, swelling, keratitis, corneal ulceration and scarring. The condition will give the subjective feeling of a foreign body in the eye. While there is generally a low rate of infectivity, the trachoma agent can be transmitted from person to person through poor personal hygiene, flies or contaminated material. At the turn of the century trachoma would be expected to run a chronic course usually progressing to serious sight loss, frequently to blindness. The first evidence of the infective nature of trachoma came in 1907 from two Austrians, Halberstaedter and von Prowazek, who had been working on conjunctival scraping from infected patients.[28] Contemporary treatment of trachoma involved a thorough but sparing removal of the trachomatous infiltration by chemical, thermal, mechanical or surgical means, while emphasis was placed on promoting eye hygiene.

Trachoma was well known in Russia, Poland and the Russian Baltic provinces, the main source of Jewish immigrants to Britain and the United States. The disease, while common, was especially associated with severely adverse economic conditions and with cold, damp and overcrowded housing. In fact, many publications of the period attest to the high incidence of trachoma in Eastern European Jews, leading many writers to conclude that there was a Jewish racial predisposition to the condition.[29] However, it was also accepted that where Jews lived in better, or at least healthier, surroundings, the incidence of the condition was no different from that of their non-Jewish neighbours. The uneven spread of the disease in European Jewry also militated against the idea of a racial predisposition. One example was the low incidence of the disease amongst the Jews of Hungary compared with Jews in the nearby Austrian province of Galicia.

The long journey across Europe meant that there might be

several opportunities for the identification of trachoma in the migrants. Travellers from Galicia might be picked up and returned home after an inspection at the Austrian-Russian border. Most health rejections were for trachoma, or other eye diseases, possibly as many as 5% of would-be emigrants. Other inspections followed at the port cities along the transmigrant routes. The diagnosis of one member of a large family travelling together might spell disaster. Having spent their entire life savings on the tickets to America, it was not usually feasible for the whole group to return home and it was often necessary for the family member with trachoma to be left behind, as in the Sholom Aleichem story quoted at the beginning of the chapter.

Trachoma in the Immigrant Population

In its Report in 1903, the Commission on Alien Immigration commented on the presence of 'granular ophthalmia' among immigrant children, but there was considerable difference of opinion amongst those giving evidence about the amount of trachoma in Jewish immigrants to Britain.[30] It was noted that there was a problem amongst some Jewish immigrants and that control of entry of patients with trachoma had to be addressed. However, other issues, such as its incidence in poorer native children, seemed to be a greater concern. Dr. Francis Tyrrell, Surgical Officer of the London Ophthalmic Hospital, took a strongly anti-alien line. He believed the Jews to be racially susceptible to the disease and claimed that his hospital was treating eighty Jewish aliens each week with granular ophthalmia, more than half of all such patients in London.[31] They were, he said, beginning to receive cases returned from America, and patients were looking for Certificates of Freedom from Infection prior to travel. Not surprisingly, he was supported by Major Evans-Gordon MP, who wished to use trachoma as a constraint on immigration.

The other medical opinions contrasted sharply with Tyrrell's evidence. The Medical Officer of Health for Manchester, Dr. James Niven, admitted to encountering only an occasional case of trachoma and said that he had not noted any particular association with the local Jewish population.[32] Dr. Niven's evidence was supported by the Medical Officer of Health for Whitechapel, the main immigrant area in London, and by Dr. Shirley Murphy who saw no need for health restrictions on immigrants.[33] William Lang, President of the Ophthalmological Society of the United Kingdom, also criticised Tyrrell's evidence.[34] He had examined 600 children at the Jews' Free School and his opinion was that the disease, while chronic, was treatable and was not one peculiar to Jews.

Indeed, an editorial in the *British Medical Journal* in April 1903 concluded that immigrant health was actually better than that of the general population and that there was not much evidence of infectious disease.[35] This finding confirms other positive contemporary reports of Jewish health patterns often attributed to family structure, religious observance and rare alcoholism.[36]

Trachoma in Glasgow

Early in 1905 the Medical Officer of Health (MOH) for Glasgow, Dr. George Wilson, published a Memorandum, based on a study by Dr. Currie, referring to a number of cases of trachoma being treated in the various ophthalmic institutions in the city.[37] According to the MOH, these patients were all aliens, as he noted that trachoma was not known to be endemic even among the poorest of the native population of Britain. He identified the aliens as either immigrants attempting to integrate into the life of Glasgow and the West of Scotland, or transmigrants who were travelling across Scotland on their way, usually, from Eastern Europe to the United States of America. Medical examiners in Glasgow were rejecting about ten transmigrants each month in Glasgow after a further eye inspection organised by the shipping companies.

There was, at any time, a significant number of emigrants waiting in Glasgow for onward travel to the United States. There could be between 400 and 500 temporarily accommodated in hostels or registered lodging houses, with the overflow in private homes, and it was often among this population that infectious disease could be found. If transmigrants were spending only a short time in Glasgow, then their trachoma might have escaped detection but cases were often identified by medical officers acting for the shipping companies and for the Marine Hospital Service of the United States.[38] However, given that patients with trachoma might be returned to their last European port if rejected at Ellis Island, it was felt important that British port cities, like Glasgow, should have a proper system for inspection and treatment.

The following record of the chaotic conditions in which immigrants with health problems were received in Glasgow illustrates the difficulties facing the authorities:

> On the evening of 26th March 1905 a Russian Jew was admitted to hospital with smallpox. He had arrived from Russia via Rotterdam and Grangemouth and was (at first) in an hotel with four others. He had visited a shop of a fellow Russian who took him to another emigrants' hotel and communicated with the medical officer of the shipping company . . . Every weekend a considerable number of emigrants are brought to Glasgow to wait for variable times before travel for the USA.[39]

It was admitted that there was no significant risk of spread of the disease, and indeed there had been no evidence of trachoma in the areas of Glasgow where the immigrants predominated or in the schools where their children were pupils. Indeed, the incidence of trachoma in Glasgow was in fact not particularly high. As might be expected, London, where the majority of Jewish immigrants to Britain had settled, had more than half of British patients[40] but the Glasgow total was considerably less than that in other cities, such as Manchester and Liverpool, which had received significant numbers of immigrants, as major centres on the English transmigrant route.[41] Only 645 cases of trachoma had been treated at the Glasgow Eye Infirmary, GEI, in the period 1895 to 1903 out of a total case load of 170,314. At the Glasgow Ophthalmic Institution Dr. Currie recorded in 1905 that he had treated seventy patients for trachoma in the previous year.[42] In 1906 there was no record in the GEI Annual Report of any cases of trachoma being treated during the year (Table 5.1).

There was a real problem for Glasgow in the containment of trachoma. While some transmigrants were being examined, there was no systematic inspection for most of the transmigrants passing through the city. Dr. Currie, writing during 1905, expressed support for the Aliens Bill, then before Parliament.[43] He welcomed the provision for the authorities to restrict the admission of infected immigrants as this would take the responsibility for public health control from the local shipping companies. The main problem concerned trachoma in so-called two-stage transmigrants, travellers settling in Glasgow for some time before onward travel to North America. They were often unaware of their condition, as they had not been medically examined prior to arrival in Britain, and were not diagnosed until they were ready for the next stage of their journey. Though constant contact with the local population, the conditions for spread of the disease were established.

Thus, a proper legal exclusion of sufferers from trachoma, 'properly a disease of the aliens', seemed to Dr. Currie to offer the opportunity to 'intercept the infective stream at its fount'. Until that time he acknowledged that local measures would have to continue despite their limited effectiveness. The agitation for alien control in Britain had been prompted by a number of different factors, social, economic and often frankly anti-Semitic. As we have seen, the use of disease control as a by-product of the legislation may have seemed prudent given the tolerable public limits of anti-Jewish expression. Major William Evans-Gordon, always ready to speak out against Jews and aliens, pointed in Parliament to trachoma, and other diseases, being introduced to Britain by alien immigrants. There were undertones of 'degeneracy', echoing the arguments of the eugenists, in much of the anti-alien propaganda.[44]

The Aliens Act restricted alien immigration to fourteen designated ports and established an inspection system for steerage passengers. Thus, despite the passage of the Aliens Act, substantial numbers of transmigrants still passed through Glasgow, some

15,576 in 1906, the first full year since the passing of the Act, with 11,991, mainly Jewish transmigrants, from Russia/Poland and Austria/Hungary.[45] Statistics for the first years after the implementation of the Aliens Act confirm that most of those refused admission to Britain were suffering from trachoma.[46] The percentage of transmigrants rejected because of trachoma was even higher, maybe reflecting the activities of some unscrupulous shipping agents in smuggling trachoma patients into Britain for treatment (Table 5.3).[47]

In 1906 the Glasgow Medical Officer of Health reported that the American Committee for Immigration was returning cases of trachoma, mostly among Jews, to Glasgow.[48] The number of cases being returned to Europe naturally increased as the medical examination at Ellis Island became more sophisticated.[49] However, the numbers sent back to Glasgow remained small, with a peak of twenty-seven cases in 1909 (Table 5.4). About half of those returned were Jewish, most being sent back to homes in Central or Eastern Europe with just a few remaining in Glasgow, usually with family. Some moved on from Glasgow to London or Leeds, while a number of Lithuanian Catholics repaired to the Lanarkshire coalfields. Factors producing a fall in numbers of those returned to Europe were the heavy financial penalties for shipping companies taking infected passengers, namely a US$100 fine per patient, the travel costs of returning the patient to Europe and the deposit guarantee with the British Government to cover onward travel.[50]

Because of trachoma's low infectivity the various measures employed by the shipping companies, in conjunction with the American Marine Hospitals Service, minimised the effect of the condition within Glasgow. In fact, it was the thoroughness with which examinations were made in Glasgow that ensured identification of the condition as a public health issue. If aliens with significant disease required treatment in Glasgow, it may have seemed better for those with milder symptoms to 'suffer in silence'.[51] In 1907 the Glasgow Eye Infirmary Report recorded that HM Inspector, appointed under the terms of the Aliens Act of

1905, had applied to the hospital secretary for a report on the prevalence of trachoma among the immigrant population of Glasgow for the purpose of a report for the Secretary of State for Scotland. While appropriate reports were compiled, none can be identified in Government archives.[52]

The Lancet noted in May 1911 that, while the third house surgeon at the Royal London Ophthalmic Hospital had treated 94 patients in one week the previous month, the introduction of the Aliens Act had made no appreciable difference to the number of cases treated in the hospital.[53] However, this might have been due to relaxation in examination procedures rather than an improvement in immigrant health.[54] Jewish philanthropy, identifying trachoma as a potential cause of anti-Semitism, helped make inroads into meeting the requirements of Jewish patients.[55]

By 1914 the issues had changed. Because of its incidence in certain city schools, and not related to Jewish immigration, Glasgow Corporation resolved to make it a notifiable disease from October 1914, under the terms of the Infectious Disease (Notification) Act of 1889.[56] In fact, Glasgow was the only British city to make trachoma a notifiable disease, and this decision was taken for purely local circumstances. Trachoma was no longer required to put a medical face on anti-alien legislation and it ceased to be recognised as a specifically immigrant problem within a few years of the passage of the Aliens Act. Indeed, from 1910, reports on the functioning of the Aliens Act did not specify the medical cause of exclusion of the alien from Britain. In any case a falling proportion of those refused entry were excluded because of trachoma and more were denied access to Britain on economic grounds. The caseload at the GEI fell substantially after 1911 with more evidence of trachoma in the indigenous Glasgow population. Only 14.4% of cases notified between 1914 and 1937 in Glasgow were in alien patients, though some of those of British birth were children of aliens (Table 5.3).

In the end, the trachoma issue, which had at first been seen as a hurdle for potential Jewish immigrants to Britain, proved to be less important once the political issues around the admission of aliens had been resolved in 1905. Trachoma was monitored for a time after the Aliens Act passed into law but its significance did not match the expectations of the opponents of Jewish immigration.

TABLE 5.1. *Cases of Trachoma Treated Annually in the Glasgow Eye Infirmary*

Year	*Average Number Treated Annually*
1850–1894	35
1895–1903	72
1904–1910	99
1911–1914	47

Source: *Annual Reports of the Glasgow Eye Infirmary*

TABLE 5.2. *Cases of Trachoma Notified to Glasgow Medical Officer of Health*

Total number of cases notified between 1914 and 1937: 982

Country of birth:

Scotland	721 (73.4%)
aliens	142 (14.4%)
Ireland	94 (9.6%)
England	25 (2.6%)

Source: T S Wilson, 'The Incidence of Trachoma in Glasgow 1914–1968', *Health Bulletin*, Vol.XXVII, July 1969, p.15

TABLE 5.3A. *Numbers of Immigrants and Transmigrants Rejected under the Aliens Act (1905)*

	Immigrants rejected	*Trachoma*	*Transmigrants rejected*	*Trachoma*
1906	133	52	1419	almost all
1907	398	257	710	674
1908	250	116	266	248
1909	451	238	494	455

Source: *Lancet*, 13th May 1911, Vol.1, p.1298

TABLE 5.3B. *Numbers of Immigrants and Transmigrants Rejected under the Aliens Act (1905)*

	Immigrants Rejected	*Medical Reasons*	*Financial Reasons*
1910 (6 mths)	459	132 (28.8%)	327 (71.2%)
1911	1053	207 (19.7%)	846 (80.3%)
1912	1390	328 (23.6%)	1062 (76.4%)
1913 (6 mths)	832	115 (13.8%)	717 (86.2%)

Source: Annual Reports on Alien Immigration 1910–1913, *Parliamentary Papers*, Vols. LV, pp.805–862; LX, pp.521–559; LXIX, pp.862–873

TABLE 5.4. *Patients with Trachoma returned from USA/Canada to Glasgow*

	Number	*Jews*	*Remained in Scotland*	*Returned to Central/Eastern Europe*
1908	8	8	0	8
1909	27	14	5	9
1910	21	12	na	na
1911	8	3	0	3
1912	6	3	0	3
1913	12	4	1	3

Source: Reports of the Medical Officer of Health for Glasgow, file DTC, 7/11/3, Glasgow City Archives, Mitchell Library, Glasgow

References

1 G S Wilson, Memorandum by the Medical Officer of Health on the Presence of Trachoma in Certain Alien Immigrants, in Report of the Medical Officer of Health for Glasgow (1905), pp.130–131, file DTC 7/11/3, Glasgow City Archives, Mitchell Library, Glasgow.

2 Roy Porter, *The Greatest Benefit to Mankind: A Medical History of Humanity from Antiquity to the Present* (London, 1997), pp.639–640.

3 Karl Pearson, Margaret Moul, 'The Problem of Alien Immigration into Great Britain, Illustrated by an Examination of Russian and Polish Jewish Children', *Annals of Eugenics*, Volume 1 (1925–1926), p.2.

4 *Ibid.*, p.45.

5 Karl Pearson, Margaret Moul, *Ibid.*, *Annals of Eugenics*, Volume 3 (1928), p.254.

6 Sander Gilman, *The Jew's Body* (New York, 1991), pp.64–68.

7 John Efron, *Defenders of the Race: Jewish Doctors and Race Science in Fin-de-Siècle Europe* (Yale, 1994), pp.58–90.

8 *Ibid.*, pp.68–69.
9 *Jewish Encyclopaedia*, Volume 12 (New York, 1925), pp.293–295.
10 Gilman, *op.cit.*, p.69.
11 *Jewish Chronicle*, 14/8/1891.
12 E Yew, 'Medical Inspection of Immigrants at Ellis Island 1891–1924', *Bulletin of the New York Academy of Medicine*, Vol.56, June 1980, p.495.
13 A K Chalmers, *The Health of Glasgow 1818–1925: An Outline* (Glasgow, 1930), p.420.
14 E Yew, *op.cit.*, p.496.
15 Howard Markel, ' "The Eyes Have It": Trachoma, the Perception of Disease, the United States Public Health Service, and the American Jewish Immigration Experience, 1897–1924', *Bulletin of the History of Medicine*, Volume 74, 2000, pp.525–560.
16 Royal Commission on Alien Immigration, 1903, Volume 1, p.34.
17 Howard Markel, *op.cit.*, pp.540–542.
18 E Yew, *op.cit.*, pp.493–494.
19 A Henry, 'Among the Immigrants', *Scribner's*, March 1901, p.302, quoted in I Howe with K Libo, *The Immigrant Jews of New York: 1881 to the present* (London, 1976), p.44.
20 *Handbook of the Medical Examination of Immigrants* (Washington DC, 1903), p.7, quoted in E Yew, *op.cit.*
21 S M Aronson, 'Trachoma and Immigration', *Medicine and Health*, Rhode Island, Vol.80, March 1997, pp.76–77.
22 E Treacher Collins, Introduction, in J Boldt, *Trachoma*, trans. J H Parsons and T Snowball (London, 1904), p.xxxvi.
23 J Boldt, *op.cit.*, p.64.
24 Royal Commission on Alien Immigration, 1903, Vol.2, evidence of F E Eddis, 21713.
25 J Boldt, *op.cit.*, p.207.
26 E Treacher Collins, *op.cit.*, p.xxxv.
27 M J Al-Rifai, 'Trachoma though History', *International Ophthalmology*, p.12.
28 C H May and C Worth, *A Manual of Diseases of the Eye* revised M L Hine, (9th edition, London, 1946), p.128; Sir John H Parsons, *Diseases of the Eye*, revised H B Stallard (10th edition, London, 1947), p.177; E Treacher Collins, *op.cit.* p.xii; J Boldt, *op.cit.*, p.50.
29 Royal Commission on Alien Immigration, 1903, evidence of Dr. F A C Tyrrell, 3666.
30 Ibid., evidence of Dr. J Niven 21739, Dr F A C Tyrrell 3666, W Lang 20569, Dr. J Loane 4480.
31 Ibid., evidence of Dr. J Niven 21739.
32 Ibid., evidence of Dr. J Loane 4480; evidence of Dr. S. Murphy 4722.
33 Ibid., evidence of W Lang FRCS 20569.
34 *British Medical Journal*, editorial, 1903, Vol.2, pp.423–424.
35 D Dwork, 'Health Conditions of Immigrant Jews on the Lower East Side of New York: 1880–1914', *Medical History*, Vol.25, 1981, pp.1–40; Kenneth Collins, *Second City Jewry: the Jews of Glasgow in the Age of Expansion 1790–1919* (Glasgow, 1990), pp.163–165.
36 A K Chalmers, *op.cit.*, pp.416–422.
37 E Yew, 'Medical Inspection of Immigrants at Ellis Island', p.493.

38 Glasgow Ophthalmic Institution, Annual Report (1907), at Greater Glasgow Health Board Archives; Glasgow Eye Infirmary Minutes, GHB 3/1/4, p.351a, at Greater Glasgow Health Board Archives.
39 Royal Commission on Alien Immigration (1903), Dr F A C Tyrrell 3666.
40 Aliens Act (1905), Annual Report 1908, Parliamentary Papers, Cd4102, Vol.87, p.941.
41 Glasgow Ophthalmic Institution, Annual Report (1907).
42 Ibid.
43 Ibid.
44 B Harris, 'AntiAlienism, Health and Social reform in Late Victorian and Edwardian Britain', *Patterns of Prejudice*, Vol.31, 1997, pp.3–12.
45 Aliens Act (1905), First Annual Report, 1907, *Parliamentary Papers*, Cd3473, lxvi, 767.
46 *The Times*, 11th April, 1911.
47 *The Lancet*, editorial, 1911, Vol.1, p.1298.
48 T S Wilson, 'The Incidence of Trachoma in Glasgow 1914–1918', *Health Bulletin*, Vol.xxvii, July 1969, pp.15–17.
49 E Yew, *op.cit.*, pp.495–498.
50 Report of the Medical Officer of Health of Glasgow, 1908, p.150, file DTC 7/11/3, Glasgow City Archives, Mitchell Library, Glasgow.
51 T S Wilson, *op.cit.*
52 Personal communications from Public Record Office (Q98/12382) 26/1/1998; National Archives of Scotland (GEN) 2/10/1997: on file with author.
53 *Lancet, loc.cit.*
54 Gerry Black, Health and Medical Care of the Jewish Poor in the East End of London: 1880–1939, unpublished PhD thesis, 1987, University of Leicester.
55 Eugene C Black, *The Social Politics of Anglo-Jewry: 1880–1920* (Oxford, 1988), p.163.
56 T S Wilson, *op.cit.*, p.15–17.

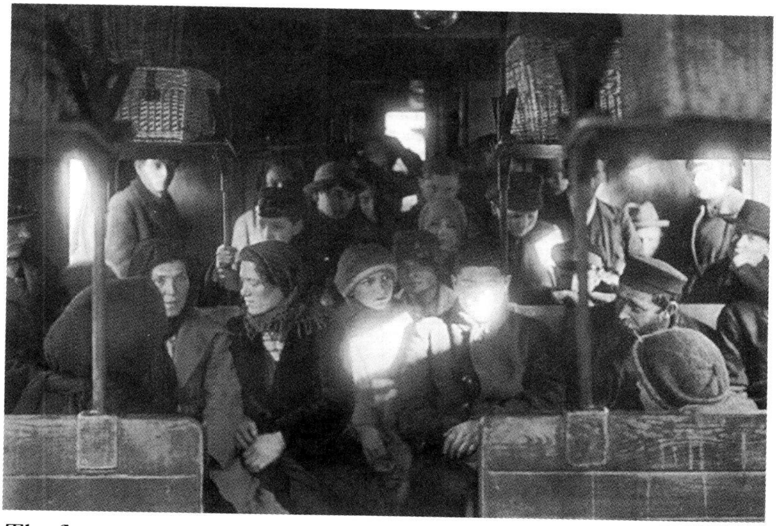

The first stage of the journey from the *shtetl.*

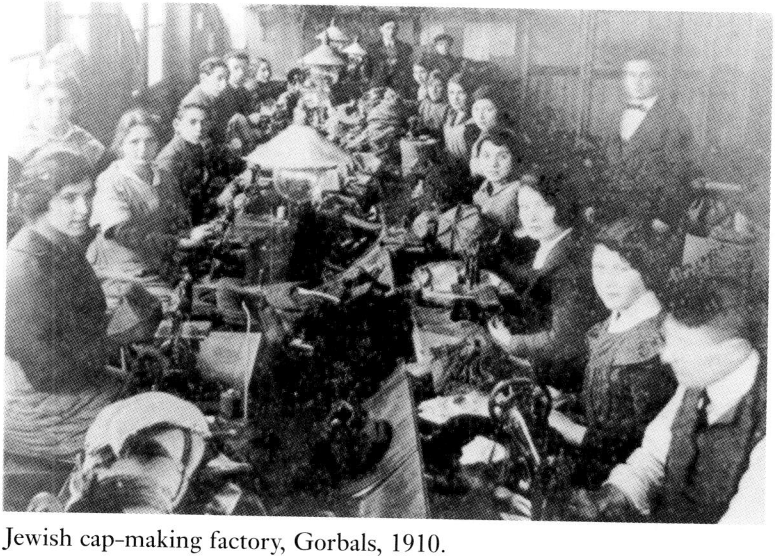

Jewish cap-making factory, Gorbals, 1910.

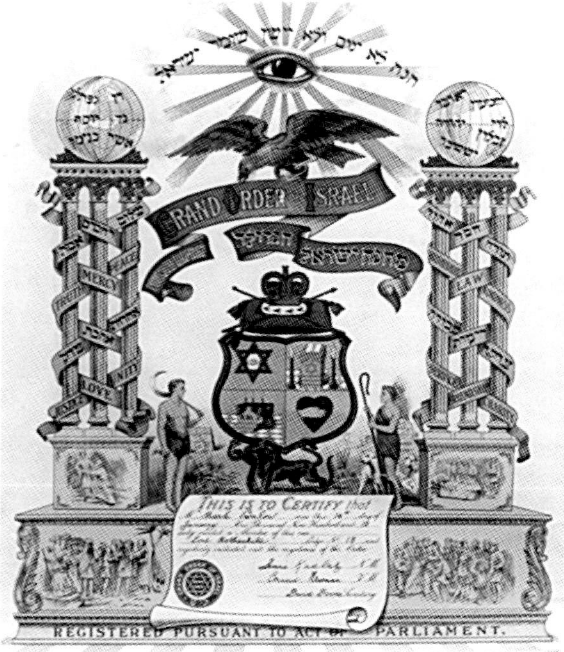

Glasgow membership certificate of Lord Rothschild Lodge, Jewish friendly society.

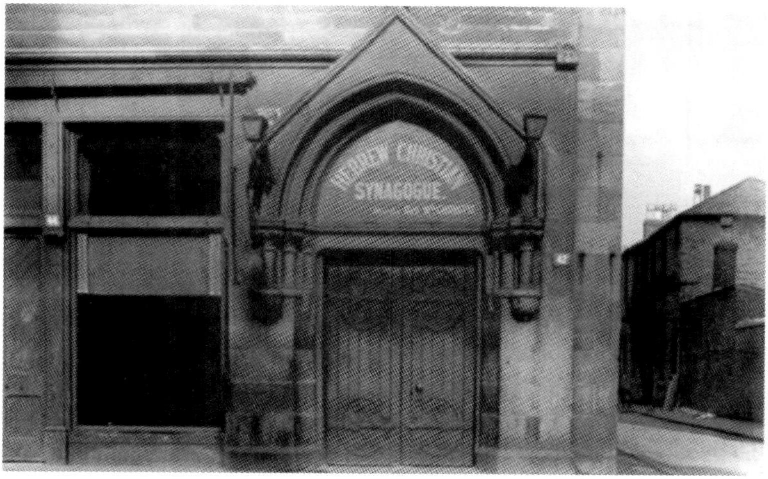

Hebrew Christian Synagogue, Gorbals. Centre of Christian missionary activity. *Glasgow City Archives.*

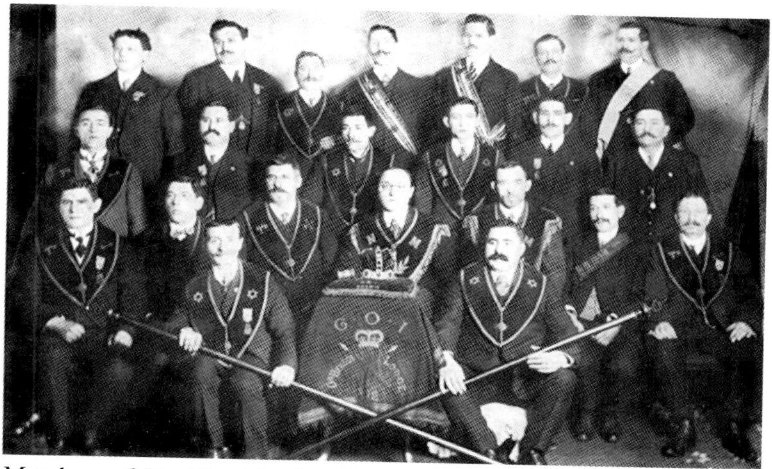

Members of Dr. Herzl Lodge, Grand Order of Israel, Jewish friendly society, Glasgow, 1905. *Scottish Jewish Archives.*

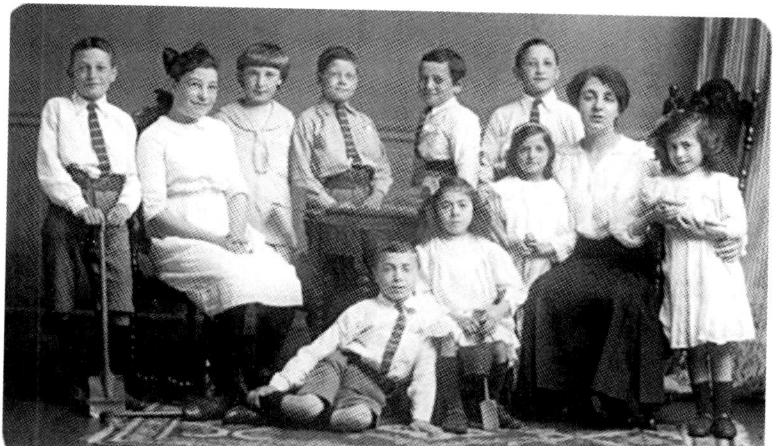

Matron and children at the Gertrude Jacobson Orphanage, Glasgow, 1917. *Scottish Jewish Archives.*

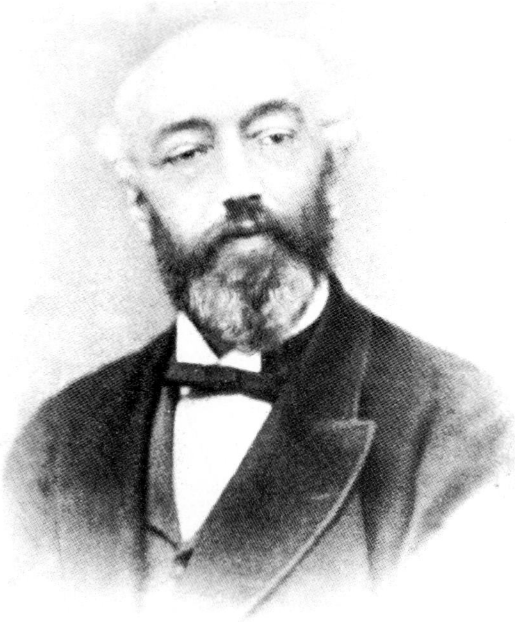

Dr. Asher Asher.

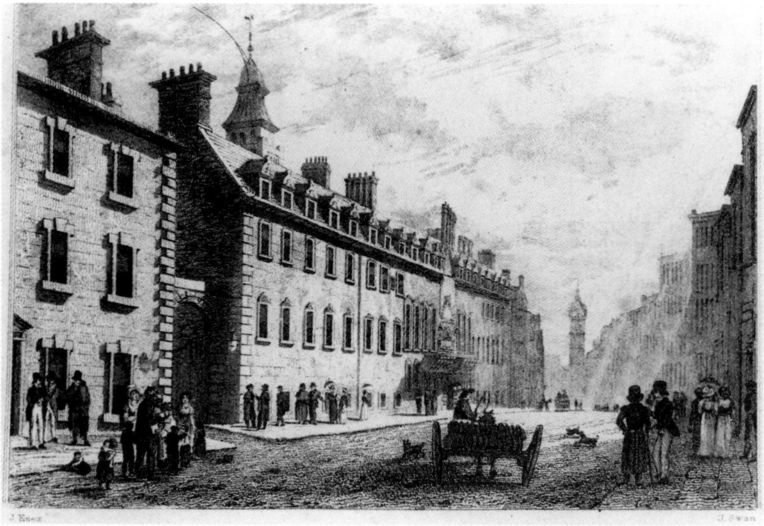

University of Glasgow, High Street, early nineteenth century.

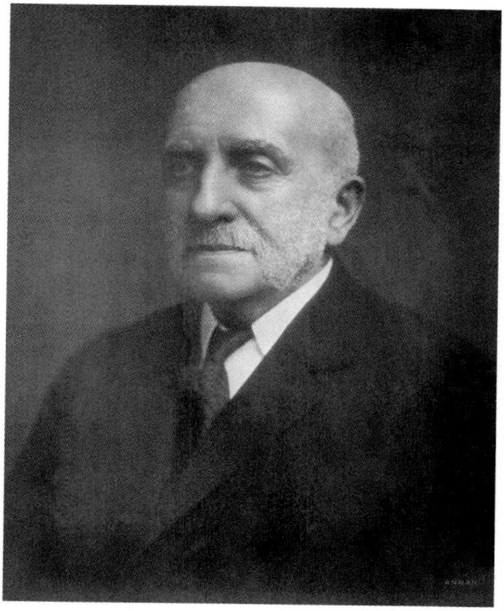

Joseph Fox, Chairman, Glasgow Jewish Dispensary. *Scottish Jewish Archives.*

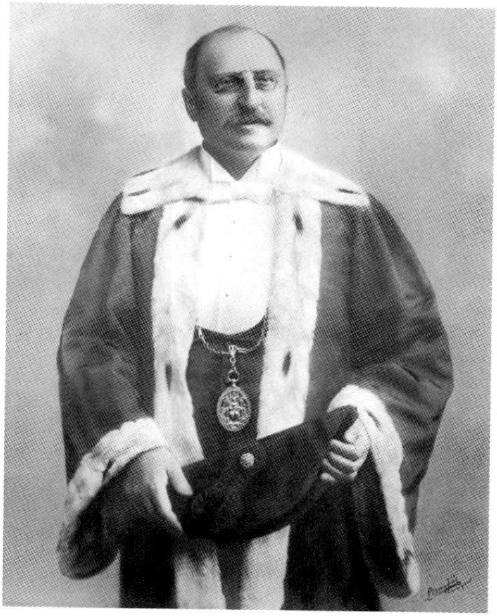

Bailie Michael Simons. *Scottish Jewish Archives.*

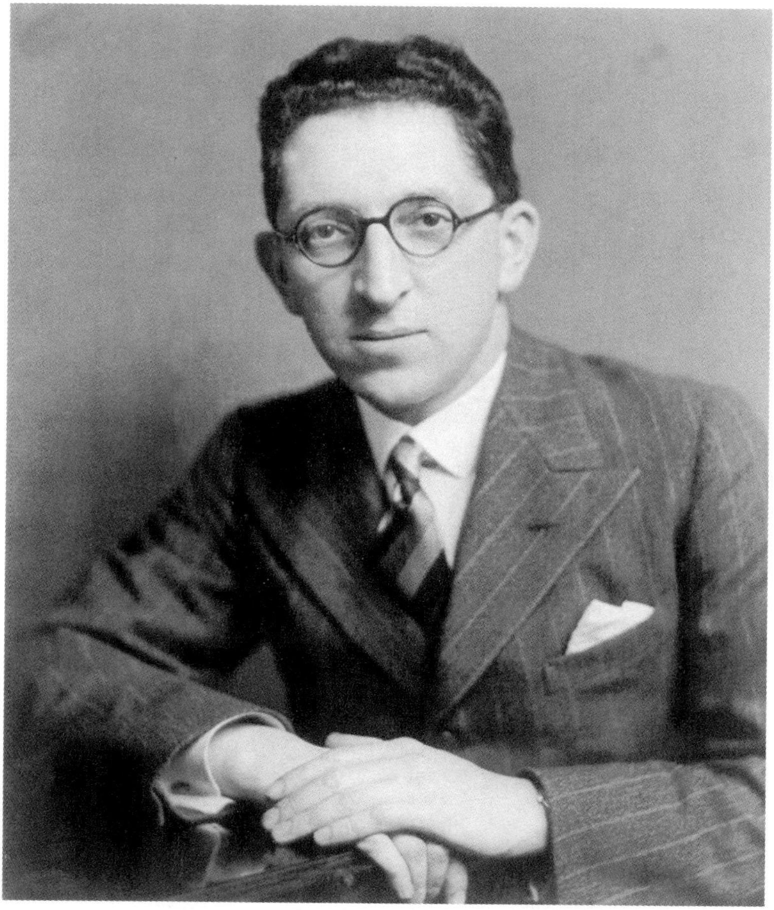

Noah Morris, the first Glasgow Jew to become Regius Professor of Materia Medica at the University of Glasgow in 1937.

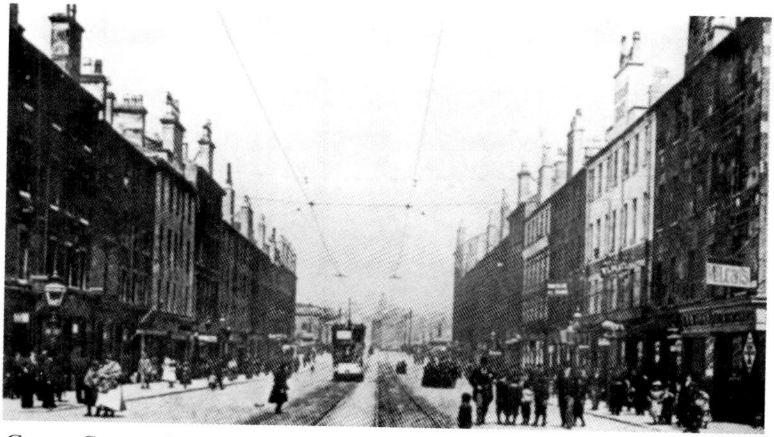

Crown Street, Gorbals. Some Gorbals streets were wide and airy with a prosperous appearance.

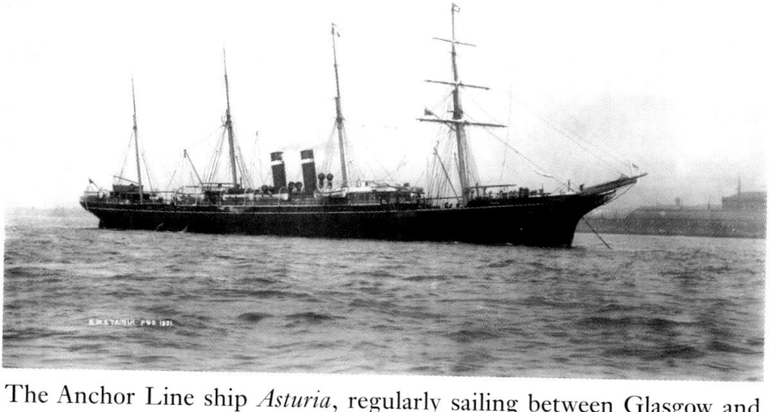

The Anchor Line ship *Asturia*, regularly sailing between Glasgow and New York, 1900.

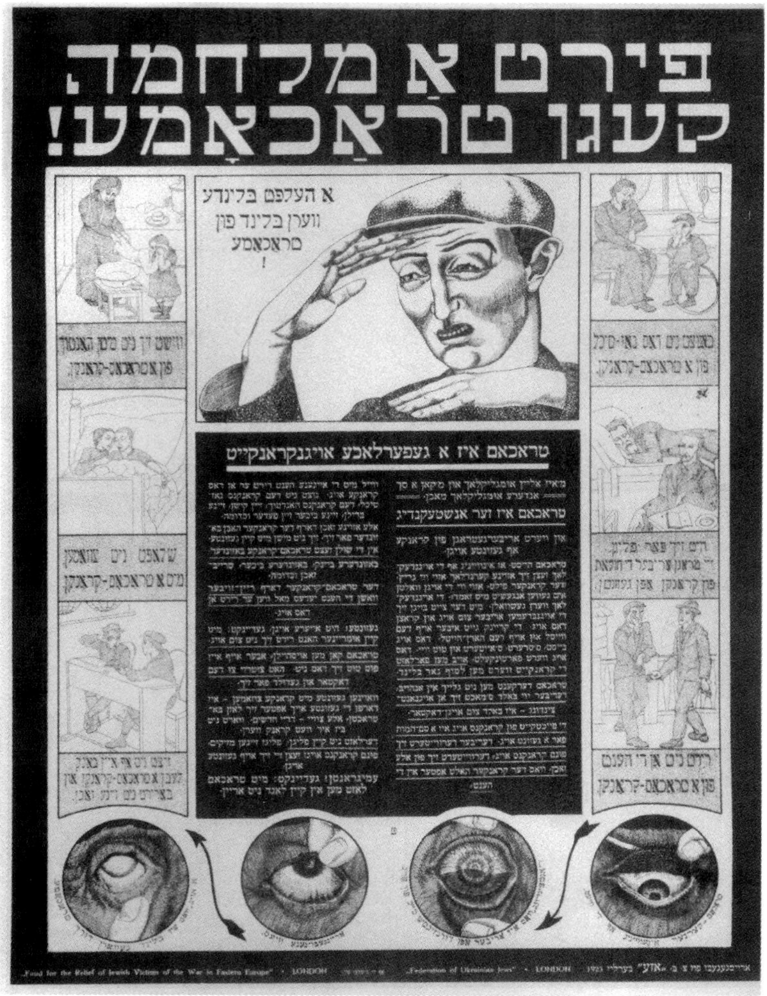
פירט אַ מלחמה
קעגן טראַכאַמע!
א העלפט בלינדע
ווערן בלינד פון
טראכאמע
!
טראכאם איז א געפערלאכע אויגנקראנקייט
טראכאם איז דער אנשטעקנדיג
„Fund for the Relief of Jewish Victims of the War in Eastern Europe" • LONDON
„Federation of Ukrainian Jews" • LONDON

Immigrants were examined for trachoma, as this poster shoes, at Ellis Island, New York. *Yivo Institute for Jewish Research, New York.*

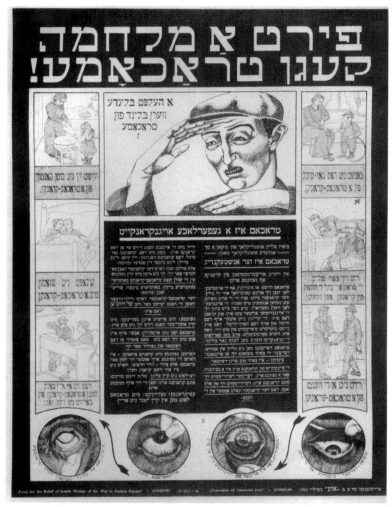

CHAPTER SIX

Mental Health

'Patient is extremely restless and noisy and as ill-behaved as only a Jew can be'.
From patient case-history, Govan District Asylum, 1910

'Patient is a Russian, speaks English imperfectly and is unable to give any account of himself . . . little information can be obtained from his friends on account of their limited knowledge of English'.
From patient case-history, Govan District Asylum, 1905

Population dislocations, especially those of economic and political refugees, are often said to be associated with mental health problems. There is often pressure, sometimes subtle but occasionally more obvious, on immigrants to acculturate quickly to the norms of the host society. Immigrants tend to develop the same kind of psychological problems as both their family 'back home' and their new neighbours.[1] Immigrants, suspicious of life around them, may develop persecutory delusions though these are not necessarily specific to them, or they may find that their own behaviour patterns are labelled as disorders by their new host society.[2] In fact as Littlewood and Lipsedge point out, 'to discuss the psychological adjustment of ethnic minorities is to underline yet again the popular conception of them as a problem'.[3]

It is possibly significant that the term alien, thus far in this book applied only to the Jewish immigrants to Britain, can also be applied to lunatics: two different elements, both potentially adrift from society's mainstream. While there was evidence given to the Royal Commission on Alien Immigration that many of the newcomers came with a strong sense of purpose aiming at self-improvement,[4] there is equally the possibility that many of those who move homes and countries do so because of an inability to fit easily into the society around them. The Jewish newcomers settled more easily in Glasgow because there was a familiar Jewish religious and cultural milieu that had been faithfully reproduced in Scotland. However, many of those who wished to leave the *shtetl* travelled no further than the growing Polish or Baltic cities of Dvinsk, Lodz or Warsaw[5] where the wider cultural environment was better known and where Jews formed a larger proportion of the population.

During the nineteenth century Jews were said to be particularly predisposed to mental illness, or at least prone to hospitalisation in the great urban centres where Jewish communities were concentrated. In London there was said to be an increased Jewish incidence of hysteria, neurasthenia and melancholia.[6] We have seen how, with tuberculosis and trachoma, racial theories were proposed to account for the Jewish incidence of these conditions. Anthropologists like Georg Buschan could point to Jewish racial identity as cause for raised or lowered incidence of disease. Quoting 'four to six times higher rate of mental illness' in the absence of alcoholism pointed to, he believed, an inherited weakness of the central nervous system.[7] Various theories, whether racial or religious, based on Jewish endogamy or degeneracy were adduced. Some saw a Jewish link between the attribute of genius and the prevalence of mental illness, both over-represented in nineteenth-century Jewry. Jewish creativity was thus associated with Jewish madness.[8]

Gilman has clearly illustrated the European belief in the Jewish predisposition especially to hysteria and neurasthenia, quoting, for example, Jean Martin Charcot, whose views that 'nervous illnesses of all types are innumerably more frequent among Jews than among other groups' quickly became commonplace in European psychiatry.[9]

Jewish communal organisations believed that Jews had a greater risk of mental illness. In 1873 the Jewish community in Britain was urged to try to find out why this was so, but in fact this was a common theme of different communities in many countries in the years of Jewish mass migrations.[10] The newly arrived immigrant Jew was obviously most at risk while the accultured, emancipated Western Jews sought to distance themselves from the link with Jewish madness. Jewish preoccupations with mental illness during the nineteenth century formed part of an increasing awareness of the problems posed by health problems that actually can be traced back to ancient times. As mental illness was being diagnosed, more asylums were being built all over Europe.[11] In Scotland, following earlier developments in England, the Scottish Lunacy Act of 1857, which set up the Scottish Lunacy Board, was a catalyst for reform.[12]

In Glasgow, the only provision for the mentally ill was in the parish poorhouses and the Glasgow Asylum, based at Gartnavel since 1843. Govan District, where from the 1890s most of Glasgow's Jewish community lived, relied on accommodation in its poorhouse while sending some patients to Greenock or Gartnavel.[13] The 180-bed Govan Parochial Asylum at Merryflatts, now the site of the Southern General Hospital, was opened in 1873 with thirty acres of ground.[14] Within a few years Merryflatts, despite a large extension taking the capacity to 244, was overcrowded and the now independent Govan District Lunacy Board acquired a new site at Hawkhead for building on a larger scale. Known as the Govan District Asylum, though since 1964 called Leverndale Hospital, one of its main catchment areas included the Gorbals.

The Govan District Asylum opened in 1895 with capacity for 424 patients, 280 of whom were in the asylum and 144 in the hospital wing, increasing to 520 patients in 1908. Between 1890 and 1918 there were 67 Jewish admissions at the Govan District Asylum out of a total of 5,750 (1.2%). Smaller numbers of Jewish patients, but in a similar proportion, were to be found in the Govan Parochial Asylum used mainly for admission and assessment prior to transfer to Hawkhead. A few Jewish psychiatric patients were also treated at Gartnavel Royal Infirmary in Glasgow's West End and at Crichton Royal Infirmary in Dumfries, in the south of Scotland.

In this chapter we will look at the hospitalisation of Jewish patients for mental ill health in Glasgow between 1890 and 1914, using hospital admission records and case-notes. Religion of all admissions to psychiatric hospitals was recorded in the Admission Ledgers and thus identification of Jewish patients was easily established. With this information we can examine the attitudes of examining physicians to the Jewish patients and analyse the additional pressures placed on patients by factors related to ethnicity, physical ill health and family dislocation.

Similar findings in regard to language, food, delusions and doctors' attitudes to Jewish patients were identified in a study of Jews in psychiatric institutions in Liverpool, Birmingham and Manchester in the third quarter of the nineteenth century.[15] Smith's study, published just a little over a year after the first presentation of these Glasgow Jewish psychiatric case histories, confirms the importance of looking at whether the manner of the reception of Jewish patients, with their religious and ethnic behaviour patterns, could be seen as part of the disorder itself.

Case Records

For the period studied case records were kept in large bound ledgers that could contain the notes of hundreds of patients. The notes were recorded by hand and had details of the patient, including age, height and weight besides an outline of the medical and psychiatric history on admission. Patient testimony was usually recorded in the second person along with the doctor's opinion of value of the patient's evidence. The records were regularly updated, although in chronic cases this might become quite infrequent, with changes in the mental and physical condition of the patient, and indicated outcome details, such as whether the patient was discharged, either cured or still unwell. If the patient died, the cause of death was usually recorded. The Lunacy Commission inspected the records twice a year and laxity could be censured.

Record-keeping in asylums was an invention of the nineteenth century. Gradually the role of note-keeping was extended, often for medico-legal reasons as well as with the aim of improving patient care.[16] Case notes at asylums during this time tended be rather conservative laws unto themselves.[17] Andrews has noted that one can often learn more about the preoccupations of the medical regime in the asylum than about the patients and their stories. He showed that the information they contain can provide an illuminating insight for the medical historian, as 'far from representing patients' impressions, case notes pre-eminently constitute the impressions of the medical officers who wrote them'.[18]

Records were rarely kept to a standardised format although the Govan records studied did have a framework which allowed quicker recording of the basic data, a device often used to allow the psychiatrist more time for the interesting clinical work.[19] It was not just immigrant Jewish patients and their families who might have difficulties in the encounter with the psychiatrist taking a clinical history. Families were often reticent about divulging sensitive information, especially if they thought that the family name might be stigmatised.[20] Doctors could also be dismissive of information that they thought to be erroneous or coming from 'ignorant' informants. With language problems these difficulties could be greatly exaggerated.

Medical staff at Govan tended to be Glasgow graduates who went on to medical careers in other Glasgow hospitals.[21] Most junior doctors stayed only a few years although those appointed to more senior positions served on average as Medical Officer for about eleven years. One of the leading figures at the Govan Poorhouse and Asylum during the main period of Jewish immigration to Glasgow was William Watson. Watson was Resident Medical Officer during the 1870s and, after a brief spell at Barony, was appointed as Medical Officer in 1883, finally serving as Medical Superintendent of the Govan District Asylum from 1894 until 1913. It was only during this last period that Glasgow medical graduates would have learned some psychiatry as undergraduates as mental disease teaching became a requirement for the MB ChB examination in 1889, and the course was made compulsory in 1892.[22]

Language Problems

For a new immigrant community the English language itself was a major problem. Glasgow had from 1888 English language classes for the Yiddish-speaking newcomers organised jointly by Glasgow Corporation and the Jewish Literary Society. Providing English classes fell neatly within the ambit of the Literary Society which had been established in 1888 to anglicise the newcomers and provide a synthesis of Jewish and British cultural life.[23] As we shall see, lack of ease in English was one of the primary motivating factors for the opening of a Jewish Dispensary in the Gorbals as late as 1912 in competition with Christian missionary groups who employed a Yiddish-speaking apostate doctor in an attempt to lure Jewish patients into the mission halls.[24]

In the Gorbals, the proliferation of Jewish welfare and self-help organisations gave more opportunities for Jewish patients to receive services that closely matched their ethnic needs. For psychiatric patients who were new immigrants the difficulties were compounded. Jewish patients had to contend with a hostile environment where there were unfamiliar sounds and non-kosher food. They were separated from family and friends and from the facilities of the Jewish community. Usually they were the only Jewish patient on the ward. Further, with the emphasis placed on history taking in psychiatry, the difficulty in obtaining a clear account of the illness often prevented doctors from making adequate assessments and from prescribing treatments from the meagre resources then available.

It was not always possible to obtain a proper account of the illness from relatives and friends, who themselves were likely to have been recent immigrants and faced with the same problems. There were few Jewish doctors in Glasgow before the First World War, and so non-Jewish doctors almost invariably admitted Jewish patients for psychiatric care. Indeed, it was only once recorded that a Jewish doctor, Dr. A.A. Finkelstein, who for a time around 1895–1898 held the official position of Medical Officer to the Glasgow Jewish Board of Guardians, admitted a Jewish patient to the hospital.

The following are some records of language-related problems extracted from patients' case records:

> Deluded and self absorbed – resents being paid attention to as she is unable to speak English that she can be understood.[25]

> . . . more depressed possibly arising from the reason that no one can speak to her.[26]

> Her ignorance of English makes it difficult to say if she is incoherent or not.[27]

> He seems to be delusional but owing to his imperfect knowledge of English the nature of his delusions is unclear.[28]

> Patient is a Russian, speaks English imperfectly and is unable to give any account of himself . . . little information can be obtained from his friends on account of their limited knowledge of English.[29]

As time went on it was more likely that members of the Jewish community would have become more acculturated with a greater command of the English language. From 1912, while there were still many Jewish patients with language difficulties, it could be recorded:

> She speaks Yiddish as a rule and English occasionally.[30]

> She is a Russian Jewess but speaks English fairly well.[31]

> She speaks little English but it is possible to get some information from her in German.[32]

Although Jewish immigration to Britain declined after the passage of the Aliens' Act in 1905, there was still a steady and significant immigration of Jews from Eastern Europe to Britain up to the outbreak of the First World War. Thus, even after the beginning of the War it was still being recorded of a patient that 'mental state is difficult to estimate correctly – patient is a Russian and has been in Britain only a year – linguistic difficulties'.[33]

Tuberculosis

As we have seen, the problem of pauper consumptives posed considerable difficulties for the Jewish welfare services in Glasgow. Tuberculosis was a particular problem within the mental illness institutions. It was frequently encountered in the debilitated psychiatric patient or in another member of the family and was often the cause of premature death in the asylums:

> Sleepless at night, delusional, not caring for her 7 children. Husband suffers from TB and spent 18 months abroad being treated. He is now often off work. She appears in consequence to have undergone considerable provocation and to have had an undue amount of domestic worry.[34]

> Physically he is reduced, poorly nourished and shows signs of phthisis pulmonalis. He has had two haemoptyses, sweats at night and has a hacking cough.[35]

Family Separation and Migration

The period of Jewish migration at the turn of the century was characterised by considerable family dislocations. Often, the breadwinner left Russia or Poland first, later sending for the family as financial circumstances permitted. When physical and mental illness were present, this clearly presented additional stresses to family members, with an isolated individual in one country and maybe a wife and children waiting patiently, often in financial difficulties, elsewhere. Illness for any member of families in transit whether physical or psychiatric could be one further factor in prolonging family separation.

In Britain immigrants with mental ill health could be deported if within one year of arrival they had been 'found wandering without ostensible means of subsistence'.[36] In major illnesses which have natural remissions and relapses dockside diagnoses, except in the most florid of patients, would not likely be successful. In America those campaigning for restrictions on immigration claimed that insanity in the newcomers was a threat to society.[37] This claim was not taken seriously until the first years of the twentieth century. However, even into the twentieth century mental health analysts could point out that the immigrant population did not have any undue excess of psychiatric problems. While immigration policy was to restrict entry of insane immigrants, there were continuing problems with effective inspection and control at the ports of entry. The second case quoted here illustrates the ability of the American authorities to return psychiatric patients across the Atlantic to their last port of embarkation:

> Domestic worry owing to husband's absence in America and she has little to live on. No family history can be obtained.[38]

> About 1911 the patient went to New York to join her husband who had emigrated there some 9 months previously. About a week after she arrived she became suspicious of her husband's mother who lived in the same house and even blamed her for putting poison in her food. In consequence, the husband rented another house for himself and his wife. For some time she was more contented but complained of heart beatings when her mother in law was present and complained that she had thrown powder into the air about her. She then showed neglect of her duties and the children. She cut her throat with her husband's razor and was removed to Long Island State Hospital in Brooklyn and deported to Britain.[39]

> Two previous episodes of mental illness and married previously in Russia.[40]

There are also recorded instances of Jewish patients from Glasgow visiting Russia before returning, in ill health, to Scotland. For example, it was noted of one patient that he 'speaks English fairly well but with a foreign accent. Went to Russia two years ago and was later expelled so came to this country. Says that when he was in Polish Russia he wandered about doing nothing'.[41]

Food Problems

The provision of kosher food for Jewish patients in Glasgow hospitals was a major preoccupation of the Glasgow Jewish community. It was 1913 before an arrangement was made with Merryflatts for a kosher kitchen to be established. There are no indications in these records of psychiatric patients being provided with kosher meals, or of there being any particular difficulty with Jewish patients taking the regular meals. Such references as there are to food are as likely to relate to the kind of problems that any patient in a psychiatric institution of the period might face. However, it is hard to believe that for Jewish patients, or their families, in the immigrant period the dietary laws would not be accorded prime importance although it has to be accepted that in the climate of nineteenth-century psychiatric institutions any deviance from the accepted behaviour could risk delaying discharge. Rev. Green, a visitor to Jewish asylum patients in the London area, spoke about the pressure on these patients to eat *treifa*, considering that the lack of kosher food provision could impede patient recovery.[42] The following are examples recorded of Jewish patient food refusal:

> Refused to eat his dinner, as he wants to leave room for the food his father is bringing him today.[43]
>
> She has not been taking her food well sometimes refusing it altogether.[44]

Jewish Attitudes and Anti-Semitism

Anti-Semitism has a pervasive presence in Western culture in different times and places. This prejudice is based on ideas of alien race and language and, as Gilman has shown, extends to stereotyped attitudes to perceived Jewish physical defectiveness. Thus, hearing a 'Jewish' accent or voice may provoke anti-Semitism and the Jewish body, even the 'Jewish' foot, may represent both the physical otherliness of the Jew to the anti-Semite with an inherent, even diabolical, disability.[45] Thus, some case records report the following descriptions of patients:

> She has the features of a Jewess.[46]
>
> In her incoherent talk she shows the Jewish hatred of Christians.[47]
>
> Undersized and presents various signs of physical degeneracy.[48]

One patient was described as 'Ape faced little woman . . . A most excited specimen of the race of Israel. Jabbers constantly in an uncouth guttural tongue'.[49] However, just a few weeks later she had recovered a little, but enough to be 'communicative and speak freely on her religion'.[50] Another less than flattering patient description was the following:

> Belongs to Russia and gives his birth-place there . . . His huge mouth and large teeth together with his shifty eyes give him a very evil appearance. Patient is extremely restless and noisy and as ill behaved as only a Jew can be . . . Frequently asks if the questioner is a Jew or gentile.[51]

Delusional Symptoms

With mental illness manifested as delusions of persecution mention of the United States was not uncommon, often the favoured ultimate destination of many Jewish immigrants to Glasgow. Many immigrants saw themselves rather as transmigrants with the journey through Scotland, arranged by enterprising Scottish shipping lines, only as an opportunity to make a little money and learn some English before arrival in *di goldene medine* across the Atlantic. Of one patient it was recorded that 'he had certain enemies who were trying to do him harm they had prevented him obtaining work in this country and in America'.[52]

The nature and content of delusion symptoms can be an indication of the culture and history of the period. Many patients, clearly paranoid, believed that they were victims of plots and conspiracies and that those in attendance were ranged against them. Again, language and cultural differences could exaggerate these fears. Given the more religious climate a century ago, some patients had delusions about God while others reflected more immediate political concerns:

> . . . imagines God speaking to him . . .[53]

> . . . emotional, noisy and conversing with his father in heaven . . .[54]

It was recorded of one patient that he 'thinks he is the Kaiser'[55] but exactly one year later he 'never has anything to say for himself and is demented. He never speaks of his being the Kaiser now'.[56]

Family Support

Despite the opening of the first Jewish residential institutions in Glasgow just before the First World War, the focus of Jewish care in Glasgow was definitely the home. However, the cramped conditions of many newcomers, in squalid subdivided apartments in the Gorbals tenements, were not conducive to the care of the mentally disturbed. There are records of patients being hospitalised only as a last resort and of patients being removed from hospital and taken home when they were really far from recovery:

> Difficult to form a precise opinion as regards this patient's mental condition as she cannot speak a word of English and so her notions are unknown to us. Her friends, however, state that she still has absurd ideas and they cannot undertake to look after her. Her general conduct and manner confirm this idea.[57]

In the case of one seriously ill patient it was recorded that 'her friends have removed her in order to place her under treatment in another institution. She is demented, impulsive and dangerous'.[58] Given the seriousness of her condition and the level of care required to care for her, it was recorded that her removal was 'a miracle'. LW, a 20–year-old message boy with 'hallucinations and delusions', was discharged unimproved back to the care of his mother in the Gorbals in June 1910.[59] AK, a 43-year-old with insomnia, delusions of grandeur and persecution with visual and auditory hallucinations, was only admitted after his wife in Norfolk Court in the Gorbals had been coping with his symptoms for five months.[60]

Treatment Outcomes

Of forty-one patients in whom long-term outcomes could be determined, about twenty were discharged home, either 'recovered', or in a condition which family or friends could reasonably cope with. Nine died in hospital, three from tuberculosis and six from other causes, while a further twelve remained in long-term care whether in the Govan District Asylum or in other institutions around Scotland. In one or two cases recovery seemed spectacular:

> Improved greatly – he is almost well again. Patient converses readily and most intelligently. He speaks several languages fluently and is thoroughly acquainted with current political topics in Russia and Germany.[61]

ML was allowed out of hospital on the 29th of March 1913 after earlier in the month attempting suicide using a hatpin. However, he had only managed to pierce the skin over his heart. Three months later in June 1913 the *Glasgow Herald* carried a story that he had attacked his stepmother with nitric acid and afterwards had committed suicide by cutting his throat.[62]

These excerpts from the case histories of Jewish patients in the Glasgow psychiatric hospitals give a flavour of contemporary Jewish life and of attitudes to Jewish patients by the doctor recording the case histories. Mental illness was a tragedy in Victorian times and it was especially so for Jewish patients. As immigrants in a new country, unfamiliar with language, diet and even the basic asylum regime, hospitalisation, and the uncertain attention of sometimes bewildered clinical staff, was often an unavoidable last resort.

TABLE 6.1. *Jewish patients and total admissions at the Govan District Asylum, Hawkhead Hospital, Glasgow*

Year	*Jewish patients (%)*	*Total admissions*
1895	0	66
1896	2 (1.0%)	198
1897	0	131
1898	1 (0.4%)	287
1899	2 (0.9%)	224
1900	1 (0.4%)	262
1901	3 (1.2%)	244
1902	3 (1.2%)	241
1903	1 (0.4%)	240
1904	4 (1.3%)	314
1905	2 (1.0%)	205
1906	7 (3.2%)	221
1907	4 (1.6%)	249
1908	1 (0.5%)	219
1909	2 (0.8%)	231
1910	7 (3.3%)	215
1911	2 (0.7%)	273
1912	3 (1.0%)	293
1913	5 (1.8%)	278
1914	4 (1.5%)	268
1915	5 (1.5%)	334
1916	2 (0.8%)	256
1917	5 (2.2%)	224
1918	1 (0.4%)	244
Total	67 (1.2%)	5750

Source: Extracted from Admission Ledgers of the Govan District Asylum, GGHB Archives, Mitchell Library

TABLE 6.2. *Jewish patients and total admissions at Govan Parochial Asylum*

Year	*Jewish patients (%)*	*Total admissions*
1895–1899	4 (1.1%)	369
1900–1904	2 (1.1%)	174
1905–1909	2 (1.2%)	165
Total	8 (1.1%)	708

Source: Extracted from Admission Ledgers of the Govan Parochial Asylum, GGHB Archives, Mitchell Library

References

1 Roland Littlewood, Maurice Lipsedge, *Aliens and Alienists: Ethnic Minorities and Psychiatry,* 2nd edition (London, 1993), p.86.
2 *Ibid.*, pp.87–88.
3 *Ibid.*, p.xiii.
4 Interdepartmental Committee on Physical Deterioration, PP, 1904, Vol.XXXII, Part 2, Cd2210, Evidence of Dr. A K Chalmers, Q6090.
5 Stephen D Corrsin, 'Aspects of Population Change and of Acculturation in Jewish Warsaw at the end of the Nineteenth Century: the Censuses of 1882 and 1897', in Wladyslaw T Bartoszewski, Anthony Polonsky, eds., *The Jews in Warsaw: A History* (Oxford,1991), pp.212–231.
6 Gerry Black, Health and Medical Care of the Jewish Poor in the East End of London, 1880–1939, unpublished PhD thesis, University of Leicester, 1987 p.34.
7 Sander L Gilman, *Smart Jews: the Construction of the Image of Jewish Superior Intelligence* (Lincoln, 1996), p.169.
8 Sander Gilman, *The Jew's Body* (New York, 1991), pp.132–133.
9 Sander L Gilman, *Love + Marriage = Death, and other Essays on Representing the Difference* (Stanford, 1998), p.99.
10 *Ibid.*, p.104; *Jewish Chronicle*, 5/12/1873.
11 Frank Rice, 'Care and Treatment of the Mentally Ill', in Olive Checkland, Margaret Lamb, eds., *Health Care as Social History: the Glasgow Case* (Aberdeen, 1982), p.59.
12 Jonathan Andrews, "*They're in the Trade . . . of Lunacy, They 'cannot interfere' – they say. The Scottish Lunacy Commissioners and Lunacy Reform in Nineteenth-Century Scotland* (London, 1998), pp.16–17.
13 Jonathan Andrews, 'A failure to flourish? David Yellowlees and the Glasgow School of Psychiatry: Part 1', *History of Psychiatry*, viii, 1997, p.186.
14 *Ibid.*, p.187.
15 Leonard D Smith, 'Insanity and Ethnicity: Jews in the Mid-Victorian Lunatic Asylum', in *Jewish Culture and History*, Vol.1, 1998, pp.27–40.
16 Jonathan Andrews, 'Case Notes, Case Histories, and the Patients' Experience of Insanity at Gartnavel Royal Asylum, Glasgow, in the Nineteenth Century', in *Social History of Medicine,* Vol.11, pp.256–259.
17 *Ibid.*, p.261.
18 *Ibid.*, p.265.
19 *Ibid.*, p.261.
20 *Ibid.,* p.263.
21 Jonathan Andrews, 'A failure to flourish? David Yellowlees and the Glasgow School of Psychiatry: Part 1', *History of Psychiatry*, viii, 1997, p.195.
22 Jonathan Andrews, 'A failure to flourish? David Yellowlees and the Glasgow School of Psychiatry: Part 2', *History of Psychiatry*, viii, 1997, p.333.
23 Kenneth Collins, *Second City Jewry: the Jews of Glasgow in the Age of Expansion: 1790–1919* (Glasgow, 1990), p.70.
24 *Ibid.*, pp.158–159.
25 HB/SH/1/4/1899.
26 HB/AA/14/2/1901.

27 HB/GF/10/10/1918.
28 HB/JC/8/6/1903.
29 HB/JS/8/6/1905.
30 HB/ET/6/8/1912.
31 HB/TMC/16/9/1916.
32 HB/GF/29/9/1915.
33 HB/AK/3/12/1914.
34 HB/TMC/16/9/1916.
35 CR/FS/31/5/1894.
36 *Jewish Chronicle*, 24/6/1910.
37 Gerald N Grob, *Mental Illness and American Society 1875–1940* (Princeton, 1983), pp.169–171.
38 HB/ES/26/2/1914.
39 HB/ET/6/8/1912.
40 HB/AK/3/12/1914.
41 CR/LB/30/11/1891.
42 *Jewish Chronicle*, 9/3/1877; 22/2/1878.
43 HB/SM/23/7/1916.
44 HB/FC/16/5/1902.
45 Sandor Gilman, *The Jew's Body* (New York, 1991), pp.3–5.
46 HB/ET/6/8/12.
47 HB/FG/8/4/1916.
48 HB/RV/31/12/1908.
49 CR/HB/22/4/1893.
50 CR/HB/5/5/1893.
51 HB/HA/22/8/1910.
52 HB/LL/23/7/1904.
53 HB/SS/28/8/1902.
54 HB/AN/1/5/1905.
55 HB/HG/22/9/1914.
56 HB/HG/22/9/1915.
57 HB/AA/17/6/1902.
58 HB/CF/9/6/1911.
59 HB/LW/1/6/1910.
60 HB/AK/3/12/1914.
61 HB/JG/15/6/1910.
62 *Glasgow Herald*, 6/6/1913.

Case notes are designated by file, patient initials and date. Patient records from Govan District Asylum records are in ledgers HB 24/5/1–36 while Govan Parochial Asylum records are in ledgers HB 17/2/136–138, GGHB Archives. CR: patient records at Crichton Royal Infirmary, Dumfries.

CHAPTER 7

Jews in Medicine

'. . . the combination of a thoroughly religious God-fearing spirit with scientific accuracy.'
Chief Rabbi Dr. Nathan Adler, describing Asher Asher, from Notes and Correspondence of Asher Asher, 14/3/1872, in Hartley Library, University of Southampton

'Among Jews, medicine and faith have always been intermingled and it is difficult to establish where the one finishes and the other begins.'
Chaim Bermant, *The Jews* (London, 1979), p.138

Jewish Medical Students and Graduates in Scotland

Scottish medicine proved to be receptive to the Jewish immigrants whose obsession with health included the determination by increasing numbers to enter the medical profession. There was a significant element, which saw in medicine the road to social advancement in keeping with the Scottish tradition of the democratic ideal in education.[1] Jewish doctors, like their Scottish colleagues, achieved social advancement by medical qualification, through individual ambition and collective effort. Conditions were being set for the upward mobility of general practitioners within the medical profession despite the control over the profession wielded by an elite determined to maintain their own social status.[2]

The first Jews to enter medicine established a trend within the community and reasserted the Jewish interest in medicine so that Jewish physicians in Britain formed part of the long chain of Jewish medical tradition. In Scotland this was epitomised by the career of Asher Asher, born to poor immigrants in Glasgow, who became a successful doctor and communal leader. Asher's career still forms part of Glasgow Jewry's folk legacy and was a powerful stimulus to his later co-religionists who wished to follow the same path.[3]

The entry of Jews into medicine in Britain followed the arrival of Jews from the Iberian Peninsula and Central Europe during the eighteenth century. Unable to achieve medical education or qualifications from the English universities, some turned to Scotland to further their ambitions. There had been complete freedom of conscience in the Scottish universities, certainly from the beginning of the eighteenth century, when medical faculties began to be formed in the Scottish universities, while religious tests were still operative in Oxford and Cambridge.[4] This meant that Jews, Catholics and others could not matriculate or graduate at the ancient English universities without taking an oath of allegiance to the articles of the Church of England. Although only a small number of Jewish students and graduates can be identified in Scotland between the re-establishment of a Jewish community in London in 1656, and the eve of the great Jewish immigration into Britain from 1880, these figures must be set against the small size of the British Jewish community and its precarious status as a predominantly immigrant group. For the first generation of immigrants the overwhelming priority was always economic survival but there was a parental expectation among the Jewish working classes that their ambitious hopes for their children would be translated into real career opportunities.

The first Jewish medical students in Scotland date from 1767 in Edinburgh but Jews had been graduating in medicine in Aberdeen for almost thirty years before that. These Aberdeen degrees, awarded to existing medical practitioners on the basis of affidavits from established physicians, enhanced medical prestige and provided the stamp of British legitimacy to foreign practitioners settling in Britain. However, by the nineteenth century the practice of awarding degrees *in absentia* in Aberdeen and St. Andrews was at an end and Jewish students seeking medical degrees in Scotland were to be found enrolled in regular medical studies, usually in Edinburgh, but also in Glasgow.

The first Scottish Jews to study medicine were based in

Edinburgh and included the flamboyant chiropodist Heyman Lion (c1760–1825), Louis Ashenheim (1816–1858), later to practise in Jamaica, and his younger brother Charles (1828–1866) who emigrated to New South Wales.[5] The first Jewish medical graduates in Glasgow were Levy Myers from South Carolina who graduated in 1787 after undergraduate study in Edinburgh and Laurence Joseph who graduated in 1831 and was later known as Joseph Laurence. However, it was with Asher Asher that a Jewish tradition of medical study in Scotland began, and his path was to be followed by increasing numbers of young Jewish men in later decades as the Jewish community in Glasgow expanded and scholarships became available to support their study.

Asher Asher

Asher Asher was born in Glasgow in 1837, the first son of Philip and Hannah Asher who were both Jewish immigrants to Britain. Philip came from a rabbinic family in the Polish town of Lublin while Hannah's family were Dutch Jews.[6] The Ashers moved from London to Glasgow, then home only to a few dozen Jews, attracted by the business prospects in the rapidly expanding city. From an early age Asher was an assiduous scholar, of both Jewish and secular subjects. He was educated at St. Enoch's Parish School and at the High School of Glasgow, entering the University of Glasgow to study medicine in 1853 while only 16 years old.

Medicine would have seemed to offer a bright young man, like Asher, an alternative to his father's work in the fur trade. Yet entry into professional life for a young Jew in mid-nineteenth century Britain was not without risk. The average member of the medical profession in Glasgow was conscious of a low estimate of his worth in the city's strongly commercial atmosphere.[7] Emigration to the West Indies or Australia, following the Ashenheim brothers from Edinburgh, was a popular option. Asher would have had little contact with established practitioners, and the local Jewish community was too small to provide him with a base for a career.

Asher pursued his medical studies with enthusiasm. He had a successful undergraduate career, winning several class prizes, notably in *materia medica* and the practice of medicine. He came first in the forensic medicine class, while supporting himself during his studies with work as a bookkeeper in a local clothing firm. He graduated MD in 1856, the first Jew born in Glasgow to achieve this distinction and only the fourth Jew to have graduated at the University of Glasgow. Asher was a contemporary of the great Scottish Victorian public health specialist Dr. James Burn Russell, and their careers had interesting parallels. Both were born in 1837 and they were pupils together at the High School of Glasgow. Russell entered medicine later than Asher, completing an arts degree first, going on to become a visionary and innovative Medical Officer of Health in Glasgow between 1872 and 1898. During these years Russell promoted health policies, just as Asher did, based on improvements in housing and sanitation and the prevention of infection.[8]

After graduation, Asher became a licentiate of the Royal College of Surgeons of Edinburgh and entered work as a parochial medical officer, covering a population of 5,000 in Wester Cadder at Bishopbriggs, then a small mining town near Glasgow. There was a tradition in the Glasgow area of providing medical services for the poor, and these offered the doctor an opportunity to gain experience before progressing to another medical appointment.[9] As a young medical graduate, only nineteen years old, Asher could not have been too choosy. The salary was low, and the work, of necessity, arduous, and the Parochial Boards closely scrutinised the work of their medical officers. The job was not likely to be a sinecure though the Board might presume that an impressionable young graduate might adhere closely to their policy of financial stringency. His duties were to attend to the poor of the district, and those resident within five miles of it, without charge. Any fee for paupers, resident outwith the district, was only earned with the consent of the parochial board. Wester Cadder's annual health costs were only £20 a year, with £5 being paid to the Glasgow Royal Infirmary to cover hospitalisation of Cadder residents.[10]

To augment his meagre annual income of only £15 per year, Asher undertook private medical work in Glasgow, though he was always ready to treat those in financial need without charge. Without such private work most doctors in mid-Victorian Glasgow could not have survived financially.[11] Besides his professional activities Asher was deeply involved in the affairs of the local Jewish community, by then comprising 200 souls. From 1858 he served as the medical officer to the Glasgow Hebrew Philanthropic Society, attending the Jewish poor and sick. He was Honorary Secretary of the Glasgow Hebrew Congregation from 1860 to 1862 yet he still found time to pursue his studies in Hebrew language and Jewish religious lore. Asher exhibited a deep erudition in his Jewish studies in which he had been almost entirely self-taught.

Asher resigned his post in Cadder in December 1861 after he and his fellow medical officer in Easter Cadder had applied unsuccessfully for an increase in salary.[12] The four years in Bishopbriggs proved to be a valuable start to his career. Asher had learned well the medical and social needs of the poor and the difficulties of providing medical care with severe financial constraints. He left Glasgow for London in 1862, joining Dr. Jacob Canstatt in practice, at 4 Castle Street in Houndsditch, providing primary medical care for the Jewish poor of London. At first this care was under the auspices of some of the larger London synagogues. During 1862 the system of delivery of health care to the Jewish poor was altered with the 'Jewish Board of Guardians for the Relief of the Jewish Poor', originally founded in 1859, taking over this responsibility. Asher's medical experience, his Jewish knowledge as well as his fluency in English, Hebrew and Yiddish would have been considerable assets in his new work. He was now working for a better funded, locally based and religiously sensitive care body albeit with a reputation for patronising and parsimonious leadership. He was there at the start of its operations and showed in his work that he possessed the ability to create and develop institutions and had the vision necessary to drive forward the new organisation, recognised in the 1860s as among the most progressive philanthropic organisations in England.[13]

Asher's meticulous annual reports for the London Jewish Board of Guardians (LJBG) clearly demonstrate his care and devotion in tending to the medical needs of the Jewish poor in London.[14] (Table7.1). He provided careful guidelines for his work, providing ample statistics to permit evaluation of his activities. Canstatt and Asher received considerable financial support from the management, enabling them to carry out their work without constraints imposed by lack of medical necessities. In his first Annual Report Asher identified the key factors such as malnutrition, poor housing and a lack of sanitation which adversely affected the health of the community.[15] He made strenuous efforts to overcome the problems of lack of food and clothing, lack of cleaning facilities, poor ventilation and light and overcrowding. Convalescent care was organised, coal, blankets and cleaning materials provided and a pride in hygiene manifested. In 1865 Asher warned about the possibility of a cholera epidemic, as well as increasing risks of death from dysentery and bronchitis. The LJBG were mobilised to institute a number of sanitary measures such as drainage, water supply and lime wash. In addition a number of insanitary cellars used for housing were removed, the worst tenements were boarded up and street refuse was not allowed to accumulate to the same extent. Fevers tended to spread rapidly in the Jewish community where there was reluctance, for religious reasons, to enter the Fevers Hospital. However, the severest cases were admitted to hospital, keeping the number of deaths at a lower level.

Perhaps the key to Asher's early success was in his ensuring that the LJBG was the leading Jewish agency in the fight against the contemporary health scourges. By the time of his death as improvements in sanitation led to reduction in epidemics of cholera and typhus the Board led the fight against tuberculosis in the Jewish community. This policy extended to similar bodies round the country as Boards of Guardians, like that in Glasgow, gained credit for the contribution they made to the lower Jewish death rate from TB.[16] Asher left this medical work in 1866 after winning a keenly contested election for the post of Secretary to the Great Synagogue in London. A letter in the *Jewish Chronicle* just before the election said that it 'seemed a thousand pities to attract Dr. Asher from a profession which he adorns and in which he has shown his value'.[17]

In 1870, with the formation of the United Synagogue, linking the main orthodox synagogues in London, Asher became its first secretary. Despite his new work as a communal official Asher continued to work tirelessly for the Jewish poor. He used his new position of communal power and, above all influence, through membership on a variety of committees dealing with medical and social matters, to affect policy on a wide range of health and welfare issues. The Jewish United Synagogue Act of 1870 gave the new body responsibility for Jewish poor relief and it was some time before this was transferred to the London Jewish Board of Guardians. As late as 1885 the United Synagogue Visitation Committee Relief Fund proposed improvements in Jewish health care by setting up an organised system of lecturers and health visitors. These visitors would instruct immigrants in health and hygiene, and provide an introduction to life in London while enabling visitors to check hygiene in the home and its immediate surroundings.[18]

In an age when the average doctor needed an economic sideline to survive, Asher's transformation into a communal civil servant allowed his talents of medical organisation and support to flourish. Asher's position with the United Synagogue was well paid. His final annual salary was £700, about three times that of a Medical Officer of the LJBG a decade or so earlier.[19] Asher used his connections within the United Synagogue and the LJBG to further his interests in wider communal philanthropy. He worked closely with Samuel Montagu, who had links with the LJBG, and the Rothschild family, who were involved in the lay leadership of the United Synagogue. He travelled to Russia, America and the Holy Land, fearlessly giving advice on ameliorating the lot of Jewish immigrants and making accurate assessments of their needs. After Asher's visit to Jerusalem with Samuel Montagu in 1875, he wrote a report on conditions in the Holy City for the Moses Montefiore Testimonial Fund, set up to mark the great philanthropist's 90th birthday. This report was credited with affecting improvements in the physical situation of the Jews there though it was bitterly criticised within the religiously traditional community, known as the Old *Yishuv*, because of its emphasis on secular education.[20]

In 1882, when Jewish refugees started flooding out of Russia, Asher was appointed one of the Trustees of the Mansion House Fund set up with the contributions raised in London, under the patronage of the Lord Mayor, for Russian Jewish refugee relief. It was quickly decided to set up a fact-finding mission to Brody where large numbers of Jews were gathering at the rail junction on the Russian-Galician frontier. Asher brought some order into the chaos, providing help for all the refugees. His knowledge of Yiddish and medicine was of great value when he helped screen the thousands of Jewish refugees from Russia pouring through London, sometimes working through the night. In 1884 he visited areas of Jewish settlement in North America, gathering information about the final destination of the refugees. In 1886 he again accompanied Samuel Montagu, this time on a trip to Russia. Asher was able to pay a visit to his father's hometown of Lublin and was shocked by the conditions experienced by his relations there. Unfortunately, he developed an episode of pleurisy there, a forerunner of the lung cancer that was to end his life prematurely.

Asher took a special interest in the *Chevrat Hakneset Brit*, the society responsible for circumcising the sons of the Jewish poor. A *mohel* himself, he believed strongly that doctors should perform the rite of circumcision. He published a monograph on circumcision, *mila*, dealing at length with the religious and historical aspects of the rite, describing it as 'the foundation stone on which rests the whole Jewish polity'.[21] Asher saw moral as well as religious and national factors in the performance of *mila*, the physical means for 'arriving at moral perfection and purity'. However, by 1873, when his booklet was published, the rite of circumcision and some of its associated rituals had come under attack, especially from those who saw open anti-Semitism as unacceptable and based their antagonism to Jewish religious practice on medical, hygienic and even aesthetic grounds. Even within early radical Reform there was little enthusiasm to abrogate circumcision. Much of the opposition to circumcision centred on the performance of *metsitsa* (suction) orally.[22] Asher believed that the reasons given in the Talmud and religious codes for oral *metsitsa* were not theological but scientific and therefore concluded that the arguments should be considered from a scientific and not a theological point of view.

Asher's attitude to *metsitsa* thus set him against the Chief Rabbi, Nathan Adler, spiritual authority for the United Synagogue, as well as the London Beth Din. In compiling his book, *The Jewish Rite of Circumcision*, Asher was keen to have the approbation of the Chief Rabbi and included a number of modifications in the text at Dr. Adler's suggestion. While Adler 'admired the combination of a thoroughly religious God fearing spirit with scientific accuracy which pervades it', he was forced to write that he could not 'agree with your views on *metsitsa*'.[23] When the book eventually appeared, despite incorporating many of Dr. Adler's suggestions, it did not carry the approbation of the Chief Rabbi for anything other than Asher's translation of the laws of circumcision.[24]

Asher also clashed with the Chief Rabbi on the subject of early burials in 1873, when he proposed a delay of forty-eight hours between death and interment. Claims had been laid before the Council of the United Synagogue 'that several persons at different periods had been buried alive'.[25] The Council had ascertained that the Jewish poor were exerting pressure for the issue of a death certificate, often telling doctors that the death had occurred many hours earlier. Doctors in turn were said to be accepting the evidence of Watchers, employed by the Burial Society, without any further checking. Asher wrote to the Chief Rabbi that 'modern science has demonstrated that there is no absolute test of death but decomposition'.

Jewish law favours burial of the dead as soon as possible after death, and the formal week of mourning begins only after interment has occurred. Thus any delay in burial, especially over the Sabbath, could lead to financial hardship by extending the time required off work for the mourning rituals. Reforming Jewish physicians in Germany, concerned that members of Jewish burial societies might be unable to determine the signs of death accurately, expressed their opposition to speedy burials.[26] However, more traditional Jewish doctors were able to support traditional practice on hygienic grounds and could point to a report by the Berlin College of Medicine that early burials could reduce the spread of certain contagious diseases. In his reply the Chief Rabbi emphasised the importance of speedy burial and suggested a proper system of certification of death and of mortuary provision.[27] This would enable bodies to be removed from poor and cramped homes as quickly as possible, and particularly before the Sabbath.

Asher's critique of circumcision and early burial supported those who advocated the modification of religious practice while still operating within religious law. Asher saw no separation between religion and society. He was concerned to remove superstition from Judaism but gave support to that ideology which in the Jewish Enlightenment saw Jewish life divided into religious and secular areas.[28] Asher was thus a complex religious figure. It was not surprising, therefore, that the Chief Rabbi Dr. Herman Adler should note, in giving a sermon after Asher's death, that Asher had 'given expression to some opinions and conjectures from which I would dissent'.[29]

Thus Asher combined strict adherence to religious practice with a considerable freedom of thought. His tact, diplomacy and understanding of the views of others were legendary. Blessed with an encyclopaedic brain, his Jewish learning encompassed the full range of rabbinic literature. He wrote extensively on Jewish life and practice in the *Jewish Chronicle*, never afraid of propounding controversial views, though using a variety of aliases. His death at the early age of 51 years from lung cancer was widely mourned, not least in his native Glasgow where a marble memorial plaque was erected in his memory at the Garnethill Synagogue, and a Gold Medal and Prize was instituted at the University of Glasgow classes in diseases of the ear, nose and throat. Thus, Asher's name remains deeply respected in Glasgow and London.

He had set communal policy for health and welfare and for the co-ordination of the work of religious bodies, always displaying loyalty to his religion and community. The new waves of Jewish refugees from Russia in the years after Asher's death, with their complex social and religious needs, were easily assimilated into the framework which Asher had done so much to establish. His obituary in the *Jewish Chronicle* remarked that Asher exemplified the union of thought combined with practice in the noble tradition of the great Jewish physician Maimonides.[30] His memory remains a blessing in Glasgow where his legacy of communal service, Jewish learning and medical practice provided inspiration for subsequent generations of young Glasgows Jews seeking educational and social advancement.

The Levenston Family

After Asher the best known Jewish medical family in Victorian Glasgow were the Levenstons, who had long been settled in England, where Michael Jacob Levenston (1799–1864) had been born. His youngest son Henry was also born in England, in 1837, and it is thought that they moved first to Edinburgh before settling in Glasgow.[31] The Levenston family were probably all involved initially in the same herbalist business when Michael Jacob Levenston arrived in Glasgow with three grown-up sons, William, Solomon Alexander and Samuel, in addition to his younger sons Michael, Joseph and Henry and a daughter Sarah. Thus, the Levenstons were well represented in Glasgow by the 1850s with the first records of their activity in the city appearing in the Post Office Directories by 1852.

In that year, Dr. Samuel Levenston (1823–1914) had his home at 23 London Street, but with a business address close by in a former tobacconist's shop. Although using the title of 'Doctor', Samuel Levenston did not qualify in medicine until 1859, when he graduated MD from the University of Glasgow. Thus, he would appear to have been known as a 'doctor', even before beginning his medical studies in about 1854, as a mature student, at a time when it was not uncommon for undergraduates to enter university at the age of 16 years. This surely indicates that he began his 'medical' career in Glasgow in the family tradition of 'irregular' medical botanical practice only switching over to 'orthodox' medicine after completing his medical studies at the University of Glasgow.

In the middle of the nineteenth century, chemists and medical botanists represented a major proportion of the estimated 6,000 irregular medical practitioners in Britain, dispensing medical treatments over the counter. Medical care was often expensive and thus available only to the wealthier in society. The growing band of chemists and druggists with their middle-class status, developing professionalism and expertise set them apart from other fringe practitioners. Rich and poor often supplemented their regular medical care by resorting to unqualified practitioners drawing on traditions of folk remedies, astrology and even magical practices. An alternative was to use new sciences such as homeopathy and medical botany, sometimes supplemented by showmanship or trickery.[32]

New systems of medical botany began to appear in Britain in the middle of the nineteenth century with some based on revolutionary ideas originating in America. One such system was derived from the writings and medicines of Samuel Thomson, who made good use of cayenne pepper, steam vapour baths and lobelia to produce a therapeutic fever, arguing that 'fever' was a 'struggle of nature to throw off disease'.[33] Thomson's system, the first to revolt against orthodox medicine in the United States of America in the nineteenth century, was a great commercial success, and others were soon attracted into this growing market. In Britain, George and John Stevens of Bristol claimed to have brought over American botanic practices. John Stevens described his system in his book *Medical Reform: or Physiology and Botanic Practice for the People* and it was the emphasis on popular medicine on which the botanic practitioners relied for their success.[34] Medical reform had its British base in Nottingham but there were many adherents in Glasgow, as regular advertisements in the *Glasgow Herald* for this period show. The medical profession reacted strongly to the challenge of the new herbalists and medical botanists whose success threatened their established position. Some of this rivalry between the doctors and the medical botanists can be discerned within the Glasgow-based Levenston family whose members included both irregular and orthodox practitioners.

It must have taken some time for the separation between Samuel's herbalist past and his medical practice to be effective. Even after his graduation, his herbalist father and brothers used Samuel's surgery premises for their own activities for a while. One example of the heightened respect accorded to Samuel Levenston's decision to study medicine was the invitation, in 1858, while he was still an undergraduate, to serve as one of the three trustees for the new synagogue in Glasgow, in George Street.[35] This was the first major project of the Glasgow Hebrew Congregation, and Levenston's fellow trustees were businessmen more closely involved with the work of the Jewish community. Levenston was the only Jewish undergraduate in the city at the time as the younger Dr. Asher Asher had already completed his medical studies and, while living in Glasgow, was working in Bishopbriggs. Samuel Levenston again served as a trustee for the Glasgow Hebrew Congregation, when the new synagogue was erected at Hill Street in 1879.

In 1855, Michael Jacob Levenston opened a herbalist business under the name of Dr. M.J. Levenston at 42 Stockwell Street in the city centre. For the next decade the business was in the name of his son, listed in the Post Office Directory as Dr. William Levenston, and described as a surgeon *accoucheur*. After 1858 both Michael Jacob and William had to drop the title 'doctor'. In that year the new Medical Act regulating medical training became law and clear guidelines were laid down for the first time regarding entitlement to style oneself doctor of medicine. The *Medical Directory for Scotland* in 1856 had listed both Michael Jacob and William in a supplementary list of practitioners who had consistently failed to supply details of their qualifications. That their names fail to appear in later editions of the *Medical Directory* confirms their lack of a proper medical degree. This stripping of their veneer of assumed medical qualifications left them confirmed merely as medical botanists, and unlike Samuel, now able only to dispense herbal medication.

Solomon Alexander Levenston (1830–1887) also claimed medical qualifications to which he was not entitled. The cover of his pharmacopoeia, which he used at his business at 150 Argyle Street, Glasgow during the 1850s, describes him as Dr. A. Levenston FRCS.[36] The decision of his brother Samuel to enter the Glasgow medical school may have been affected by the prospect of an improved status and income to be derived from working as a qualified rather than as an unqualified doctor. However, in the days prior to the Medical Act of 1858, it would have been difficult for the public to differentiate between regular medical practitioners and those who claimed medical qualifications for themselves without justification. There could therefore have been some overlap in the clientele of the qualified and unqualified Levenstons, not an unlikely circumstance at a time when physicians were known to practise, free, in chemists' shops in return for a share of the profit on the dispensed medication.[37]

Solomon Levenston's pharmacopoeia listed over forty remedies for such ailments as gonorrhoea, chancre, buboes and other sexual disorders, neuralgia, nervous disability and intestinal complaints as well as treatments to prevent hair loss and to make moustaches 'luxuriant'. There were a number of general tonics, many of them based on herbal and botanic remedies. Solomon Levenston did not lay claim to have originated these preparations and credited many of them to a local medical botanist, Craufurd Muir Mackay, while others were imported from Price, Walton and Co. of Cincinnati, Ohio in the United States of America. The collection of remedies makes no mention of lobelia or steam used in medical reform but the presence of American products and American botanical ingredients such as sarsaparilla, quassia and podophyllin was obviously important. In any case we have noted that the success of the 'new' medical botanists was in their challenge to the established medical profession and in their use of a comprehensive formulary.

Solomon Levenston, now unable to pass himself off as a 'real doctor', left Glasgow to settle in Dublin in 1859, where he continued to carry on a botanical practice.[38] While Solomon's wife dealt there in second-hand clothing, Solomon Levenston gave private tuition in physiology and other medical subjects, and afterwards ran a dispensary in the High Street with a reputation for holding the patent for a cure for venereal disease. Michael Jacob soon joined his son Solomon in Dublin, living there until his death in 1864. This combination of activities, combining medical and botanic treatment with physiology, suggests that Solomon Levenston may have been involved in medical reform in Dublin. The Levenston herbalists worked in various parts of Glasgow during the 1860s with businesses in London Street, in Park Place in the West End and Nicolson Street in the Gorbals. The London Street premises were actually the site of Samuel Levenston's surgery and it was there that Henry Levenston operated his medical herbalist business for a short time. However, Samuel's use of the premises may actually have finished before Henry began business there. Medical botanists, like the Levenstons, usually derived most of their income from the poorer classes, but qualified practitioners often competed for the same business from the middle classes who wished to keep medical fees to a minimum.[39] They were often ready to try cheaper and possibly more 'promising' alternatives, which if ineffective were at least likely to be harmless.

In fact, the obtaining of a medical degree by Samuel may well have split the family, enhancing the natural competition between city doctor and medical botanists. While gaining a medical degree undoubtedly conferred additional merit on the holder, some ambitious doctors combined professional reputation-making with the promotion of specific remedies, falling back on that traditional source of income for general practitioners, the drug trade.[40] The medical profession carried on a fierce campaign during the nineteenth against fringe practice, and although they were able to push unorthodox practitioners towards the periphery of medical practice, they were unable to wipe them out.[41]

There is no evidence of great prosperity in the Levenston family in Glasgow. Both qualified and unqualified practitioners had to struggle for their livelihoods. Salaries of city general practitioners were only about £150 to £200 annually at the time while that of a parochial medical officer was a meagre £15.[42]

Indeed, the Letters Book of the Glasgow Hebrew Congregations contains frequent letters to Michael Jacob and Samuel Levenston reminding them that they are in arrears with synagogue membership contributions![43] In 1864 Samuel Levenston moved his surgery first to West Howard Street, while living in Hope Street in the city centre, later also practising there. His name disappears from the *Medical Directory* in 1881 when he was sixty years old although his surgery address was listed in the *Postal Directory* until 1906 when he would have been 85 years old. Latterly, he lived in the fashionable West End with addresses in Elmbank Crescent and Lilybank Gardens.

The Levenston connection with medical herbalism in Scotland lasted for several decades more. Joseph's son, also named Solomon Alexander Levenston (1858–1897), born in Aberdeen, practised till his death as a medical herbalist in Greenock and other places around Scotland.[44] Of all the family, only Michael Jacob and Samuel Levenston were members of the Glasgow Hebrew Congregation. In addition, Samuel was the first treasurer of the (Jewish) Masonic Lodge Montefiore when it was founded in 1888, and he had a reputation within the Jewish community for his ability to solve communal problems.[45] Samuel Levenston's medical career, the first by a Jewish doctor to be spent entirely in Scotland, commencing in medical botany and leading on to regular medical practice, illustrated the possibility of practising in both worlds though at the risk of alienating his father and brothers, who had been forced out of medical practice by their lack of qualifications. The Levenston family practitioners made no grandiose claims for their products but offered the prospect of treatment for commercial gain. With their botanical and financial opportunism they, and many other contemporary suppliers of patent medicines, formed the only serious challenge to the monopoly of the medical profession.

The practice of the Levenston family represents the integration of Jews into the commercial and professional life of the city while remaining attached to local Jewish institutions. Asher Asher and Samuel Levenston had shown that Jews could take advantage of the facilities offered for medical study, even if employment prospects led many graduates out of Scotland. For a small immigrant community the first achievements were significant enough. There were no fewer than four Scots Jewish medical graduates from the Scottish universities by 1859, at a time when there were less than 500 Jews in all of Scotland. This paved the way for developments after 1880 when, with a much larger Jewish community, the path was set for an increased Jewish penetration of the medical profession.

Jews in Medicine in Glasgow Before the First World War

The status of the medical profession in Glasgow rose steadily in the last decades of the nineteenth century as a reflection of the city's burgeoning prosperity.[46] The increased number of skilled workers created a more dependable demand for medical care which brought improvements even to those in the lower ranks of the profession. With the development of insurance society work practitioners could exchange a degree of professional freedom for a degree of security, in the form of state intervention.[47] Although many doctors were trapped in activities which carried a low salary, there were compensations such as security of employment and the chance of utilisation of the contacts made, such as on management committees, to further career prospects.[48] Hospital boards of management were increasingly attracted by an aura of success and wished to employ the best medical talent available. Nepotism and the existence of close religious or ethnic ties between doctor and patient did not disappear but there was scope for the development of achievement on merit. It is true that the majority of recruits into Scottish medicine came from the children of the middle class but there was still room for the Scottish *lad o' pairts*, and the son of the Jewish immigrant tailor. Thus the medical profession was increasingly regarded as a most desirable occupation.

The conditions were thus favourable for the entry of Scottish Jews into the medical profession. It took a few years for a group of children educated in English to develop but there are cases of students, such as Meyer Mann (Teitelmann), son of an Edinburgh cantor, entering university after only a year or two at a Scottish secondary school. The goal increasingly became a place at the medical schools in Edinburgh and Glasgow. Few of the students had private means so it was cheaper to live at home and supplement income, usually in the form of a Carnegie Trust scholarship, by additional work in such areas as teaching in the synagogue Hebrew classes or Talmud Torah.[49]

By the beginning of the First World War about twenty Scottish Jews had graduated in medicine, and the rapid growth in the number of Jews entering medicine continued in the years after the War. There was the tradition of respect that Jews had for medicine and the physician, and for the scientific and secular learning that being a doctor implied. The doctor was seen as a figure with status, both within the immigrant world and in the wider Scottish society. In addition, possession of a medical qualification was seen as a prime asset in a community only recently established after much hardship in a strange land. The strong Jewish sense of pride in the achievements of children and the willingness to make economic sacrifices were also of crucial importance.

Medicine was seen as the main professional target for Jewish students from the earliest days of Jewish entry to the universities.[50] Although there were a few arts and law students amongst the first group of organised Jewish students in Glasgow, the majority were medical. The Scottish legal profession was considered difficult to penetrate, and partnerships in the conservative law firms were hard to obtain.[51] In addition, a qualification in Scots law meant a limited geographical choice in the place of the graduate's future career. The Jewish entry into medicine in Scotland was impressive even in comparison with trends in other western countries to which Jewish emigrants had been attracted. Within one generation of the arrival of groups of destitute Jewish refugees in Scotland, never numbering more than half of one per cent of the population, with no knowledge of the English language or the mores of Scottish society, and with their Jewish ways as their common identity, a considerable professional element had emerged.

The movement of Jews into medicine in Scotland did not occur without some suspicion of prejudice or anti-Semitism, although such charges are always hard to substantiate. Jewish graduates in Glasgow felt that it was particularly difficult for them to obtain house officer posts in Glasgow's main teaching hospitals, the Royal and Western Infirmaries.[52] In the early years of the century a few Jews had obtained posts there. Palestine-born Reuben Youdelevitz-Young was appointed house officer at the Glasgow Royal Infirmary in 1906, a year after Simon Sperber, of Montreal, had become the first Jew to be appointed to the staff of the Edinburgh Royal Infirmary. A few others, but only a very gifted few, held similar posts in the main teaching Glasgow hospitals in the following years.

Most Jews saw their advancement in medicine as a means of economic and social progress while maintaining active membership of the Jewish community. For others the medical degree was the passport out of the community. Alfred Finkelstein, who had graduated at the University of Glasgow in 1895, and was the first Jew to serve as Medical Officer to the Glasgow Jewish Board of Guardians, later ceased to identify with the community.[53] The Scottish medical schools produced more doctors than Scotland's population required and there was always a regular medical emigration. The Jewish doctors qualifying in Scotland merely followed this trend, either settling in England or even going overseas. Hyam Goodman, a former pupil of Hutcheson's Grammar School in Glasgow and the first Jewish President of the Students' Representative Council of Glasgow University, graduated in 1899 and later settled in Johannesburg.[54]

There were only four Jewish doctors practising in Glasgow on the eve of the First World War. Saul Harris qualified in 1910 and was for many years the senior Jewish medical figure in the city. Harris was the first Medical Officer of the Jewish Dispensary in the Gorbals. Meyer Mann, who had qualified in Edinburgh in 1913, was for many years the Medical Officer of the Gertrude Jacobson Orphanage for Jewish Children. Simon Harry Bennett (Bloom), an extra dispensing physician at the Glasgow Royal

Infirmary, graduated in 1913 and was awarded an M.D. by the University of Glasgow in 1917 for his work on the complications of trauma and neurasthenia. Bennet, like many subsequent Glasgow Jewish graduates, had changed his surname from Bloom, believing, with good evidence, that a Jewish surname might hamper his career prospects. The fourth was Noah Morris, who had a distinguished medical career culminating in his being appointed to the Regius Chair of Materia Medica at the University of Glasgow in 1937.

Morris was awarded the Bellahouston Gold Medal, presented only for the most outstanding of MD theses, in 1921. In 1920 he was appointed Professor of Physiology at Anderson's College, one of the Glasgow extra-mural medical schools, a post he held for eight years. When he was appointed to the Regius Chair in 1937, a dinner was organised under the auspices of the Garnethill Synagogue as it was widely felt that this honour marked a further step in the integration of the Jewish community into the life of the city.[55] In fact, the community took particular pride in this appointment as Morris symbolised, just as Asher had done earlier, the successful combination of the Jewish scholar who was equally at home in the wider world.

TABLE 7.1. *Table of Diseases, Injuries & During the Year 1862 (among indoor patients)*

Diseases, Injuries &	*Total*	*Deaths*
1. ZYMOTIC DISEASES		
smallpox	99	4
measles	158	11
scarlatine	225	50
whooping cough and croup	6	2
diarrhoea and dysentery	100	9
influenza and catarrh	141	0
fevers: typhus, low, intermittent	206	5
various other zymotic diseases	76	3
2. DROPSIES, ABSCESS &	179	7
3. TUBERCULAR DISEASE	51	11
4. BRAIN, NERVES, ORGANS OF SPECIAL SENSE	54	11
5. HEART AND BLOOD VESSELS	15	6
6. LUNGS AND ORGANS OF RESPIRATION		
bronchitis	78	4
other diseases	27	2
7. STOMACH AND DIGESTIVE ORGANS		
teething	318	11
other diseases	118	0
8. KIDNEYS &	9	0
9. ORGANS OF GENERATION	28	0
10. JOINTS, BONES		
rheumatism	68	0
other diseases	8	0
11. SKIN, CELLULAR TISSUE &	43	1
12. ABORTION	13	0
13. DEBILITY	121	14
14. OLD AGE	10	0
15. VIOLENCE, SCALDS, BURNS &	13	0
TOTAL	2182	151

Source: Year Book LJBG, 1863 (compiled by Dr. A. Asher)

References

1 Charles Newman, *The Evolution of Medical Education in the Nineteenth Century* (London, 1957), pp.11–12; R D Anderson, *Education and Opportunity in Victorian Scotland* (Oxford, 1983), pp.320–321 (Table 8.11); M Jeanne Peterson, *The Medical Profession in Mid-Victorian London* (London, 1978), p.168; Kenneth Collins, *Go and Learn: the international story of the Jews and medicine in Scotland 1739–1945* (Aberdeen, 1988), pp.11–19.

2 Margaret Lamb, 'The Medical Profession', in Olive Checkland and Margaret Lamb, eds., *Health Care as Social History: the Glasgow Case* (Aberdeen, 1982), p.17.

3 Details of Asher Asher can be found in the following: Kenneth Collins, 'Asher Asher MD (1837–1889), Doctor of the Poor', *Glasgow Medicine*, 2, 1984, pp.12–14; Kenneth Collins, *Go and Learn,* pp.51–54; Kenneth Collins, *Second City Jewry: the Jews of Glasgow in the age of expansion, 1790–1919* (Glasgow, 1990), p.44; David Kohn-Zedek, *Bet Asher* (Hebrew), bound with *Asher Asher MD 1837–1889: Collected Writings* (London,1916); *The Jewish Encyclopaedia*, Vol.2 (New York, 1925), pp.180–181.

4 Kenneth Collins, *Go and Learn*, pp.11–13.

5 *Ibid*., pp.163–164.

6 David Kohn-Zedek, *Bet Asher*, pp.xii-xiv.

7 Margaret Lamb, *op. cit*., p.37.

8 Edna Robertson, *Glasgow's Doctor: James Burn Russell 1837–1910* (East Linton, 1998), especially pp.78–105.

9 Rona Gaffney, 'Poor Law Hospitals: 1845–1914', in Olive Checkland and Margaret Lamb, eds., *Health Care as Social History: the Glasgow Case* (Aberdeen, 1982), p.17.

10 Minutes of the West Cadder Parochial Medical Board, 1858–1862, GGHB Archives, Mitchell Library.

11 Margaret Lamb, *op.cit*., p.20.

12 Minutes of the West Cadder Parochial Medical Board, 1858–1862.

13 Lara Marks, *Model Mothers: Jewish Mothers and Maternity Provision in East London 1870–1939* (Oxford, 1994), p.32.

14 Annual Reports of the London Jewish Board of Guardians (LJBG), 1862–1866, MS173, Hartley Library, University of Southampton.

15 Annual Report, LJBG, 1862.

16 Annual Reports of the Glasgow Jewish Board of Guardians, 1912–1916, SJAC, Garnethill Synagogue, Glasgow.

17 Extract of letter, quoted in obituary, *Jewish Chronicle*, 11/1/1889.

18 Minutes of Visitation Committee of the United Synagogue, 18/3/1885, 2712, London Metropolitan Archives.

19 Asher's final annual salary as Secretary of the United Synagogue was £700 compared to a figure of £200 for a LJBG medical officer in the 1870s, see Minutes of Executive of the United Synagogue 1870–1902, p 394, Minutes of Executive Committee of LJBG, 1866, 1874.

20 R. Shlomo Zalman Sonnenfeld, *Guardian of Jerusalem: The Life and Times of Rabbi Yosef Chaim Sonnenfeld*, adapted by R. Hillel Danziger (New York, 1983), pp.260–261

21 Notes on Circumcision, in *Asher Asher: Collected Writings* (London, 1916), p.99.

22 *Asher Asher Collected Writings*, op.cit., p.107. For *metsitsa* see Bernard Homa, *Metzitza* (London, 1966); Jacob Katz, *Divine Law in Human Hands: Case Studies in Halakhic Flexibility* (Jerusalem, 1998), pp.320–402; Louis Jacobs, *Theology in the Responsa* (London, 1975), p.212; Immanuel Jakobovits, *Jewish Medical Ethics* (New York, 1967), pp.195–196. For an understanding of how the issue has been understood in contemporary society see Sander Gilman, *The Jew's Body* (New York, 1991), pp.93–96, 155–157; Sander Gilman, *Freud, Race and Gender* (Princeton, 1993), pp.49,65,69,86,89; Ronald Hyam, *Empire and Sexuality: the British Experience* (Manchester, 1990), pp.77–79.

23 Notes and Correspondence of Asher Asher, MS159:AS166/9, Hartley Library, University of Southampton: letters from Chief Rabbi Nathan Adler, 21/3/1872, 30/10/1872,9/12/1872.

24 See Preface in *The Jewish Rite of Circumcision with its Prayers and Appertaining Thereto translated into English with an introductory essay by Asher Asher MD* (London, 1873).

25 Statement laid before United Synagogue Council by Asher Asher, Minute Book of the United Synagogue Council 1870–1879, Vol.1, 25/4/1873, pp.195–196.

26 Ibid., response by Chief Rabbi Nathan Adler.

27 John M Efron, *Medicine and the German Jews: A History* (New Haven, 2001), pp.101–104.

28 Thomas Schlich, 'Medicalisation and Secularisation: the Jewish Ritual Bath as a Problem of Hygiene (Germany 1820s-1840s)', *Social History of Medicine*, Vol.8, 1995, pp.423–442

29 Funeral oration by Chief Rabbi Dr. Herman Adler at Bayswater Synagogue, in *Asher Asher: Collected Writings*, p.191.

30 *Jewish Chronicle*, 11/1/1889.

31 Kenneth Collins, 'Orthodoxy and Reform: Differing Practices in a Glasgow Jewish Victorian Family', *Korot: the Israel Journal of the History of Medicine and Science,* Vol.11, 1995, pp.54–65.

32 Hilary Marland, 'The Medical Activities of Mid-Nineteenth Century Chemists and Druggists, with special reference to Wakefield and Huddersfield', *Medical History*, Vol.31, 1987, p.415.

33 Samuel Thomson, *New Guide to Health* (Columbus,Ohio, 1827), pp.8–12.

34 P.S. Brown, 'Herbalists and Medical Botanists in Mid-Nineteenth Century Britain with Special Reference to Bristol', *Medical History*, 1982, Vol.26, pp.407–40.

35 Kenneth Collins, *Second City Jewry*, pp.24,27.

36 The Pharmacopeia of Dr. A. Levenston FRCS (Glasgow, unpublished, no date), copy in possession of author.

37 I S L Loudon, 'A Doctor's Cash Book; the economy of general practice in the 1830s', *Medical History*, Vol.27, 1983, pp.265–266.

38 Louis Hyman, *The Jews of Ireland: from Earliest Times to the Year 1910* (Shannon, 1972), pp.145–146.

39 Hilary Marland, *Medicine and Society in Wakefield 1780–1870* (Cambridge, 1987), p.251; David Hamilton, *The Healers: A History of Medicine in*

Scotland (Edinburgh, 1981), pp.226–7.

40 M. Jeanne Petersen, *The Medical Profession in Mid-Victorian England* (London, 1978), p.246.

41 Hilary Marland, *Medicine and Society in Wakefield 1780–1870*, p.247.

42 I S L Loudon, *op.cit.*, p.259; Kenneth Collins, 'Asher Asher: Doctor of the Poor', *Glasgow Medicine*, 2, Mar/Apr 1984, pp.12–13.

43 Letters Book of the Glasgow Hebrew Congregation 1858–1880, SJAC.

44 From Levenston family papers, letters on file with author.

45 Ibid.

46 Margaret Lamb, 'The Medical Profession', in, Olive Checkland and Margaret Lamb, eds., *Health Care as Social History: The Glasgow Case* (Aberdeen, 1982), p.17.

47 *Ibid.*, p.43.

48 M. Jeanne Peterson, *op.cit.*, p.232.

49 Kenneth Collins, *Go and Learn*, p.83.

50 Geoffrey D.M. Block, 'Jewish Students at the Universities of Great Britain and Ireland - excluding London 1936–1939', *Sociological Review*, 34 (1942), p.185.

51 *Ibid.*, p.191.

52 At the Western Infirmary there were no Jewish house officers between 1921 and 1941 out of over 700 appointments while at the Glasgow Royal Infirmary there were two Jewish house officers out of over 300 during the 1930s.

53 Kenneth Collins, *Go and Learn*, p.85.

54 *Jewish Chronicle*, 28/7/1899.

55 *Jewish Echo*, 8/7/1937.

CHAPTER 8

Jews and the Medical Missions

'This institution ought to be supported by every Jew and Jewess as it is the means of preventing many of our people from going to the missionary dispensaries where, very often, after receiving medicine for the body they get a double dose of poison for the soul.'

Joseph Fox, President, Glasgow Jewish Dispensary, *Jewish Chronicle*, 1/3/1912

One of the most contentious issues dividing Jews and Christians in the first decades of the Jewish community in Glasgow was that of Christian mission. Jews took great offence at Christian attempts to wean Jews, usually the poorest and frailest members of the community, from their faith. For the Jewish community, missionary activity symbolised hostility to the Jews by the Christian churches, which questioned the very legitimacy of Judaism in the contemporary world.[1] To Christians, evangelising the Jews was an expression of love rather than of intolerance and, increasingly, missionary groups were established with a frequency which belied the size of the Jewish community in the Christian world.

In Glasgow, and in other immigrant centres in Britain and North America, the key target of the missionary societies was the Jewish poor who were lacking financial security. Missionary groups were ready to step in to provide a wide range of medical and social benefits. Paradoxically, the increasing efforts of missionary groups in providing social, educational, and above all medical resources in the fight to win souls led to the Jewish community matching the facilities offered by the missionaries, producing a Jewish community in Glasgow that was more cohesive and better provided for than it might otherwise have been. The Jewish poor were, for the most part, able to understand the difference between the material benefits on offer and the underlying missionary message, accepting one and not the other. For their part, the missions sought to underline the value of creating good relationships with the Jewish community, as the lack of conversionist success would otherwise have deterred all but the most devoted.

The Christian response to Jews settling in Glasgow was not just the resort to mission. There were many examples of Christian support from the various Churches in response to the Jewish plight in Russia and the needs of the new immigrants in Glasgow. Christian leaders, in particular the Roman Catholic Archbishop Eyre but also including leaders of the Church of Scotland, were closely involved in support for the Glasgow efforts in raising funds for Russian Jewish relief from the earliest years of mass immigration from Eastern Europe.[2]

The first Church missions to the Jews were founded in Germany in the seventeenth and eighteenth centuries, and Scottish Christians, through the Edinburgh Society for the Promotion of Christianity to the Jews, were involved in Germany early in the nineteenth century.[3] This interest was heightened during the 1830s when the romantic notion of a specifically Scottish attempt to convert the Jews to Christianity was conceived. This Christian enthusiasm for the Jews was fuelled by messianic hopes of religious fulfilment for the gentiles, accompanied by bringing the Jews into the Christian fold. At the same time, this fervour polarised the Church where evangelicals like Andrew Bonar, in favour of mission to the Jews, showed opposition to more cautious and moderate elements. A Scottish branch of the Society for the Promotion of Christianity to the Jews was formed in 1838, fuelled by evangelic zeal, and two years later the Jewish Mission Scheme obtained formal ratification at the General Assembly of the Church of Scotland in Edinburgh.[4] Given the paucity of Jews then living in Scotland, it is not surprising that the first missions were overseas, starting in Budapest where the first missionaries were smuggled in as chaplains to the Scottish workmen on the iron bridge linking the twin cities of Buda and Pest.[5] The Church of Scotland Mission to the Jews in Budapest was not without success.

Under the leadership of 'Rabbi' John Duncan from 1841 to 1843, it attracted the scholars Alfred Edersheim and Aaron Saphir as converts. Edersheim and Saphir later studied and served as ministers in Scotland and England and in missions to the Jews abroad.[6]

The nineteenth-century Scottish missions to the Jews, in Rumania, Hungary and in the Holy Land, denoted extremes of religious commitment. They concentrated on the Holy Land where conversion had spiritual overtones of redemption and on disaffected Jews in Central Europe where baptism was described, in the words of Heinrich Heine, as 'the ticket of admission to European civilisation'. Thus missionary attention to the Jewish influx into Glasgow did not really begin until the 1890s when the level of immigration made the local Jews considerably more noticeable.

The Origins of Mission in Scotland

Within a few years of settling in the Gorbals the Jewish community faced an increasing problem with Christian missionaries trying to attract Jews away from their faith. The various missionary groups saw the presence of large Jewish groups in Glasgow and Edinburgh as a challenge. The Jewish community was the first substantial non-Christian group in Scotland, and missionary literature often referred to the presence of an alien element in Scottish life, sometimes associated with somewhat lurid language, as the following statement from the Bonar Medical Mission in 1909 indicates:

> . . . the presence of so large a Jewish community in Glasgow, (estimated to number some 7,500 souls) was a challenge to the whole Christian community of Glasgow. The invasion of our country by a large alien population was a new phase in our national life and the Church could not stand idly by if the country was to remain a Christian country.[7]

There had been missionary activity in Glasgow from 1884, which in its simplest form represented the missionary preachers at Gorbals Cross who would deliver sermons to any passers-by prepared to listen. However, missionary activities quickly became more organised and sophisticated and they were soon seen as a nuisance if not an actual threat. In Edinburgh too, Christian missionary activity developed as the numbers of Jews in the city increased. The Edinburgh Jewish Medical Mission had been founded in 1889 and in 1904, when there were about 2,000 Jews in the city, it employed the Jewish-born Leon (later Sir Leon) Levison as its missionary. Levison had arrived in Scotland in 1901 from his native Galilee and from the outset showed his interest in mission work. He was a friend of Ben Rohold, another Palestinian Jew, who worked during 1903 in the Bonar Medical Mission in Glasgow, later continuing in missionary work in Toronto and subsequently in Haifa.[8] In 1905, 1068 patients were treated at the Mission dispensary in Edinburgh, mostly newly arrived Jews who needed treatment and medical advice in Yiddish.[9]

A variety of Christian agencies, sometimes working together, occasionally in competition, but all based in the Gorbals, began to provide facilities and services for the local Jewish population. Success could not be quantified in converts. Some, like Leon Levison in Edinburgh, claimed over a hundred converts in Scotland during his thirty years of missionary efforts in Scotland, a figure hotly disputed within the Jewish community.[10] The Glasgow-based missionary, the Rev. Aaron Matthews, would refer only to 'several cases of genuine conversion'.[11] Maurice Bloch, speaking for the Jewish community in Glasgow in 1924, put the figures closer to one or two.[12] Indeed, the difficulty in obtaining any converts from mission was a universal Christian problem. Jewish audiences were at best unresponsive and could even be hostile to the Christian message.[13] A report in 1904 for the Church of Scotland Women's Association for the Christian Education of Jewesses commented that:

> . . . we have no baptisms to tell about, no startling conversions to record; but when discussions arise as to the hopelessness of missions to the Jews and questions are asked as to when decided fruit will appear we hear our ascended Lord say 'It is not for you to know the times and seasons'.[14]

Even more poignant was the death in 1893 of the Rev. Donald Urquhart, a missionary to the Jews in Glasgow, at the age of only 43 years, noted as one who 'felt greatly discouraged by his lack of success in his labours among the Jews of Glasgow'.[15]

If the missionaries were prepared to acknowledge the paucity of their converts, they attributed it to the attitudes to Christianity brought over by the Jews from Eastern Europe. The missionaries felt that the level of converts 'was not a safe test to apply', pointing out that with the Jews they were not dealing with a 'heathen' people but one with some knowledge of the Bible.[16] Nevertheless, they remained determined to continue with their efforts despite the distress, and even hostility, that their activities provoked. Dr. Macdonald Webster, Secretary of the United Free Church Jewish Committee, reported, in 1924, that:

> In our own land it is stated many Jews have come under the liberating movements of the time, and although at Glasgow, where our work has its centre, the Synagogue sets its spies and tries to intimidate those who seek to hear the Christian message, activities are pressed on with evident signs of success.[17]

Not surprisingly, such intemperate language met with a strong response both within Glasgow, and from Rabbi Daiches, rabbi in Edinburgh from 1919 and inveterate campaigner against the Edinburgh Jewish Medical Mission.

It could not, however, be denied that some Jews had converted to Christianity out of conviction. Many of these apostates were among those who were most determined to bring the 'benefits' of their new faith to their former co-religionists. Indeed, most of the Christian missionaries working in the Jewish missions in Glasgow, and in Edinburgh, were themselves Yiddish-speaking converts. This is, perhaps, not surprising, as the prospects of success, in terms of conversion, were greater in the various Scottish missions scattered around the globe. Thus, it was the Jewish apostate who was most often left to man the local mission to the Jews. Missionaries frequently operated on the fringes of both communities and often they saw themselves as occupying a neutral ground between the Jewish community and their anti-Semitic antagonists, or even as continuing to be part of both communities.[18] These missionaries tried to make their mission halls, like the Gorbals Hebrew-Christian Study House, reflect the dual nature of their background and altered convictions.

What may have started as a sincere Christian attempt to redress the wrongs done to the Jews in Russia continued as increasingly coercive attempts at conversion. No effort was made to appeal to Jewish brains for an intellectual understanding of Christianity but instead financial and welfare inducements were held out as the snare to catch the weak, sick and poorest members of the Jewish community. However, not all Christians behaved in this way. There were those in the Church of Scotland, and in the other denominations, whose motives for extending a hand of friendship were purely humanitarian.[19] Christian Hospital chaplains sought to protect Jewish patients from the well-intentioned but unwelcome missionary visits.[20] The Rev. W. Paterson, a Christian minister providing comfort to Jewish arrivals in Leith in August 1891, some of whom were in a poor physical state, commented that:

> It is hard to think that all this suffering is in the name of what is called the Christian religion in Russia . . . it was a surprising thing for them to come into contact with our Scotch Christianity, and that a Christian minister was among them to express his deep sympathy. The prayers and blessings of that great broken-hearted company were something to have.[21]

For the Roman Catholic Church Mgr. Eyre, Archbishop of Glasgow, attended the various meetings of protest about the Jewish situation in Russia and gave the Jewish community support at the highest level of the Church when it was required. On the golden jubilee of his ministry in October 1892, the Garnethill Synagogue, the Glasgow Jewish Board of Guardians and the Glasgow *Chovevei Zion* came together to present him with an

Address. They expressed gratitude that he had 'ever been animated by sentiments of the truest philanthropy and (had) at all times been ready to advance every deserving cause without consideration of race or creed'.[22]

The Glasgow United Evangelistic Association was formed in 1874 to organise, on a church-wide basis, conversionist work among the poor. It ran the Bonar Memorial Mission to the Jews from 34 Govan Street.[23] Revivalist Christian bodies were to the fore in religious life in Glasgow around the turn of the century, seeking out those estranged from Christian life. Thus, the Jews were not the only group to be targeted and indeed they were not the only non-Christian group to be sought out by evangelistic missionaries. Christian missionaries were active among the mainly Moslem Lascar sailors, of whom about 4,000 were estimated to visit Scotland each year, although Jews were the only non-Christian group settled in Glasgow.

While the Association pursued a stridently missionary path, it was also able to co-operate, possibly in the hope of improving its standing with the Jewish community when required. In December 1905, following some brutal pogroms in Russia, the Bonar Memorial Mission to the Jews issued a protest about Jewish treatment in Russia.[24] In 1908, we have already seen that a group of fifty-seven children under the auspices of the newly formed Glasgow Jewish Children Fresh Air Fund spent a week's holiday in the Association's home in the Ayrshire resort of West Kilbride, 'where every facility was given for the observance of the Jewish dietary laws'.[25]

The basic dilemma faced by the two groups was clear. For the Jews any attempt to proselytise was unacceptable, undermined the status of the community and was perceived as a threat to their existence, questioning their very legitimacy, which they were not prepared to tolerate. To those engaged in mission any attempt to oppose conversionist activity was seen as obstructive, even obscurantist.[26] For the missionaries, withdrawing from mission cut across the basis of their faith which impelled them to bear witness to their beliefs to those who were disposed, or could be persuaded, to listen. While some missionaries employed overtly brusque tactics likely to cause offence, Fred Levison, son of the Edinburgh-based missionary Leon Levison, has pointed to many instances of potential converts being held at arm's length if their change of faith would cause financial problems, for example through loss of livelihood.[27] At the same time, in a long diatribe against Rabbi Dr. Salis Daiches, Fred Levison acknowledged that Leon could be 'indiscreet' in the language he used in literature aimed at the Jewish community.

Such indiscreet language could be found in material produced for the wartime Russian Jewish Relief Fund, which raised considerable sums of money and in which Leon Levison was the key organising figure. Leading Jewish philanthropists in England and Russia initially gave their support to the Fund, though Levison's 'uncompromisingly Christian references in the fund's literature' caused the main Jewish fund involved to withdraw co-operation when Levison's committee in Edinburgh refused to drop its missionary stand.[28] The *Jewish Chronicle* opposed Levinson from the start and in an editorial entitled 'Who Has Blundered' denounced the award of a knighthood to Levinson for his work for Russian Jews as 'the prostitution of honours'.[29] In short, Leon Levison, and his colleagues in Glasgow, were out to 'win the Jew (for Christ)', and whether it was with 'only love' as opposed to 'dialogue and confrontation', the Jews of Scotland were not much interested.[30]

The Jewish Response to Mission

During the 1890s as the Jewish immigration into Glasgow began to increase, missionary activity became more noticeable. Endelman has commented that conversionist activity did not seem to be a matter of communal concern in England for the established community, pointing to a greater worry about declining synagogue attendance, increasing intermarriage and indifference to Jewish education.[31] In Glasgow the whole community was alerted to a perceived threat to the integrity of the community. In February 1894 it was felt necessary for the Jewish Literary Society, based within the established community at Garnethill and always ready to promote topics of interest, to devote a meeting to the subject. Julius Pinto, a leading member of the Garnethill community, though he had lived for many years in the Gorbals after migrating to Glasgow from Holland, suggested that 'missionaries should not be allowed access to Jewish houses and shops'. However, the most moving address was given by Rabbi Shyne, Rabbi of the Gorbals community, who spoke to the gathering in Yiddish.[32] This was an unusual departure for a Society committed ideologically to English language meetings and further confirms the great seriousness with which the subject was treated. The attendance at the meeting was such that the venue was changed at the last minute from the Society's rooms in the Garnethill Synagogue basement, which can accommodate only about 100 people, to the Synagogue itself, which has room for several times that number.

A practical outcome of this meeting was the setting up of a Missionary Vigilance Society.[33] In March 1894 the *Jewish Chronicle* congratulated Glasgow Jewry for combating the 'pernicious activities of the agents of the conversionist societies', saying that 'these gentry have been keen to discover in the misery and extremity of Russian Jews expatriated from their country a congenial and extensive field for their operations and are pursuing in Glasgow an active and aggressive policy'.[34] It was felt important within the Jewish community to give anti-missionary activity a high profile, and there are several recorded instances of specially arranged meetings to publicise this approach. On one occasion in April 1894 the Main Street Synagogue in the Gorbals was filled to hear a baptised Jew repent, in public, of his forsaking his faith and asking to be forgiven.[35] Giving the main address, Rev. E.P. Phillips said, in the course of a lengthy address, that in his long experience with missionaries no Jew had ever converted out of conviction and indeed the particular target of the missionaries were the poor, the sick and the orphaned.

The Chief Rabbi Dr. Herman Adler maintained the anti-missionary momentum, on his visit to Glasgow in May 1896. He addressed a gathering of Jews and Christians in the Garnethill

Synagogue on the subject of 'Missions to the Jews'. The fact that the Christians outnumbered the Jews present at the meeting was significant as the Chief Rabbi, not mincing his words, contrasted 'the moral degradation and depravity of the denizens of the Glasgow slums with the sober and virtuous conditions of the Jewish poor . . . the Christian task should be to raise their own lapsed masses before they attempted the conversion of others'.[36]

By the early years of the twentieth century missionary activity in Glasgow was becoming more organised. In 1900 there were two major Gorbals missionary societies, as well as a few smaller ones, specifically targeted at the Jewish community. At the time of the 1901 Census, Mauritz Michaelis, 41–year-old self-styled 'Missionary to the Jews', had served as the Missionary for the Church of Scotland Mission to the Jews, based at the Reading Rooms and Evening School at 135 Rutherglen Road in the Gorbals, for over ten years.[37] From 1898 the Glasgow Jewish Evangelical Mission, led by the Rev. Aaron Matthews and supported by a 'lady missionary', operated from the Hebrew Christian House at 12 Abbotsford Place, at the southern and more prosperous fringe of the Gorbals.[38] This House was the centre for a network of activity which included Bible classes, a night school and gospel services, especially busy on Saturday evenings when an attendance of upwards of fifty people could make the room 'uncomfortably full'.

Supporters of the mission house, which claimed 'several cases of genuine conversion', targeted Jewish homes and shops to invite Jews to the various activities and to provide their sick with medical aid and to help to secure admissions to hospital.[39] The nuisance value of these shop visits is confirmed by the complaints, made for example by the kosher butchers and poulterers, to the Glasgow United Synagogue.[40] In appealing for general Christian support for the Mission, the Rev. Fergus Ferguson of the Queens Park United Presbyterian Church commented that 'Mr. Matthews knows better than most how to conciliate and attract his own people. He knows their spirit, their nature, their prejudices as no Gentile can know them'.[41]

Other Jewish communal developments were begun as an

attempt to counteract missionary activity, which was perceived to be more sophisticated and better organised and financed. The Jewish Free Reading Rooms at 27 Oxford Street were opened in October 1900 'to counteract the evil influences of the missionaries who had similar institutions in the neighbourhood and were doing all in their power to entrap the unwary foreigners'.[42] These new Rooms were in addition to the Zionist Free Reading Rooms, which had been opened just a few months previously, in January 1900, at 38 Abbotsford Place.[43] These reading rooms provided places where Jews could meet outside poor and cramped homes and read books and journals free from the pressures of missionary activity.

Rev. E.P. Phillips confirmed that Christian missionaries were ready to finance Jewish hospital admissions in November 1900.[44] At a meeting of the Glasgow Jewish Hospital Fund and Sick Visiting Association (GJHFSVA) he spoke of his distress at the lack of support amongst the Jewish community for this organisation. The Glasgow hospitals would not arrange admissions without the appropriate 'lines' that confirmed admission rights. If the Jewish Hospital Funds, through a shortage of money, could not furnish these admission lines, the missionary societies would be quick to offer this relief as 'bait' to any Jew in need. At a public meeting of the GJHFSVA in November 1900, it was proposed that free medical treatment should be provided to Jewish patients in their own homes. At the same time it was pointed out that Jews had been slow to provide funds for lines for their co-religionists to be admitted to hospital and it was easier to obtain these from the missionaries. This clearly stimulated the Jewish community into action, and by 1911 Joseph Fox could tell the GJHFSVA that their society had provided 1500 lines of admissions for Jews to Glasgow hospitals between 1900 and 1911.[45]

The Jewish community in Garnethill were undoubtedly alarmed at the level of missionary activity and dismayed at the prospect of conversionist inroads into the large Jewish community in the Gorbals. They were well aware that poverty, disease and social isolation were widespread in Gorbals Jewry and that provision of help for these problems was the means the missionaries used to gain acceptance within the Jewish community. The provision of facilities by Christian missionaries for the Jewish community undoubtedly stimulated improvements in Jewish welfare services. Indeed, there were those in the Christian community who feared that this would be the outcome of missionary activity and predicted that better Jewish welfare would lead to an increase in Jewish immigration.[46] However, an analysis of relative resources shows that the Jewish community were more willing to fund social and welfare services than the supporters of the Christian missions to the Jews in Glasgow. In the competition for funding for the varied Scottish mission work, for the Jewish community and beyond, the Christian missionaries in Glasgow frequently bemoaned their lack of finance. In 1906 the Glasgow Hebrew Christian House admitted to a shortage of funds as increasing numbers of Jewish paupers learned to differentiate between the medical aid, which they had no problem in accepting, and the religious zeal of the missionaries, which was clearly rejected. The medical expenses of the Hebrew Christian House amounted to £181 in 1906, out of a total income of £454, a small sum compared to the joint income of the various Jewish charities and self-help friendly societies.[47] While the Glasgow Jewish Board of Guardians were struggling on an annual income of about £1,000, we have seen that poor members of the Jewish community could call on a wide range of welfare services.

In 1910, when the first World Missionary Conference was held in Edinburgh, the various Christian mission activities among Glasgow's Jewish community were brought under the sole responsibility of the Bonar Memorial Mission and the United Free Church of Scotland through a new structure known as the Jewish Mission Committee.[48] The UF Church maintained missions in Budapest, Breslau and Constantinople as well as Safed, Tiberias and Hebron in the Holy Land. The Church of Scotland, seen as representing the more moderate element within Scottish Presbyterianism and with a leadership which had, for the most part, eschewed mission for a more co-operative approach to relations with the Jewish community, still retained formal links with the Jewish Mission Committee through the traditional reports made to its Glasgow Presbytery.[49] The Rev. W. M. Christie, previously missionary to the Jews in Tiberias and Aleppo, and with special training in Jewish religious literature, was appointed missionary with Miss H. A. Allan as the lady missionary.[50]

A church hall was obtained at 46 Oxford Street to hold the usual range of prayer and study activities and the outdoor church service, in Yiddish at Gorbals Cross, was reinstated.[51] This street service, open to passers-by, sometimes spilled over into violence. Jacob Sensen, and two other missionaries to the Jews, were found guilty of causing an obstruction on the pavement while conducting a religious service one weekday evening in September 1916. Though found guilty, they were admonished and advised to desist from such meetings in the future.[52] This they did not guarantee to do as they had been conducting such services on the pavements of Gorbals Cross for almost thirty years and they clearly felt it their right to continue. A year later, in 1917, Sensen was fined 10/6 for further breach of the peace after a mêlée occurred while he was addressing a hostile crowd, and the police had to intervene to restore order.[53]

The Jewish Dispensary

With the re-organisation of Glasgow missionary facilities the Jewish community became concerned at the prospect of poor and sick Jews being enticed into well-equipped mission clinics, which were seen as a cover for conversionist activities. The Glasgow Jewish Board of Guardians, and some of the Jewish friendly societies, offered the services of a local general medical practitioner but without a dispensary where prescribed medication could be obtained. As we have seen, the Glasgow Jewish Board of Guardians, and its predecessor the Glasgow Hebrew Philanthropic Society, had retained the services of a doctor at least since 1858, when Asher Asher had been appointed as its Medical Officer. In addition, arrangements had been made with a chemist to dispense medication at cost. In London a Jewish dispensary had functioned until 1879 but had closed because of better facilities provided by local statutory health bodies. The question of re-opening a Jewish dispensary in London was considered during the 1890s precisely to counteract the operations of the London Medical Missions who considered medical work as the beginning of the proselytising process.[54] The London East Mission stated in 1912 that the sole aim of their medical work 'is to lead these people from Judaism to the light of the Gospel, and to heal the disease of the soul through curing the sickness of the body'.[55]

In September 1910 the Glasgow Jewish Hospital Fund and Sick Visiting Association convened a conference in the Bet Herzl Hall, presided over by Joseph Fox, to consider various approaches to Jewish health issues. One was the supply of kosher food to hospitalised Jewish patients, and it was agreed that the Victoria Infirmary should be approached first even though they had turned down such a request a few months previously.[56] Another was the possibility of providing a free Jewish dispensary in the Gorbals.[57] Jewish dispensaries were already in existence in other leading regional Jewish communities such as Leeds, Liverpool, Birmingham and Manchester and it seemed appropriate that one should be provided in Glasgow also. The meeting agreed that a committee should be set up to investigate the feasibility of the setting up of a dispensary whose annual costs were estimated to be about £250.

The final decision to open the dispensary was only taken in January 1911 at the same time as the Board of Guardians move from Garnethill, an important step as the new Board premises at 11 Aspley Place, in the Gorbals, was to provide much-needed accommodation for welfare and medical provision.[58] A Jewish medical student, Simon Bloom (Bennet), immediately questioned the need for such a dispensary, given the availability of care from dispensaries attached to the major city teaching hospitals.[59] A Jewish Gorbals dispensary could, he felt, lead to Jewish patients getting poorer medical care than was available at the Royal or Western Infirmaries. Bloom suggested that Yiddish-speaking patients could take an interpreter to the clinics if unfamiliarity with English was the problem and he pointed to the existence of a medical officer paid by the Board of Guardians. Bloom believed that the Mission Hall had an 'insignificant, if not altogether negligible impetus in provoking the establishment of such an institution as the medical mission hall is a perfectly harmless agency not inimical to our communal integrity here'.[60]

Joseph Fox, as President of the Jewish Dispensary, immediately criticised Bloom's attitude. If the missionaries were providing Yiddish language medical consultations and dispensing medication to the Jewish poor in the Gorbals in their mission halls, then the proposed Jewish dispensary should not be compared to facilities at the Royal and Western Infirmaries.[61] Fox commented that though the Jewish Board of Guardians did employ a prescribing physician, he did not have a dispensary, and many Jewish patients would take their prescriptions straight from the Board of Guardians doctor to the Christian dispensary!

Dr. Saul Harris, a recent Jewish medical graduate from the University of Glasgow, was appointed Medical Officer at the Jewish Dispensary and the clinic was open initially at the Jewish Board of Guardians' new premises in Apsley Place, on Tuesdays and Thursdays from 5pm till 7pm and on Sunday afternoons from 4pm till 6pm.[62] The Dispensary proved to be popular from the start and additional facilities were added later in larger accommodation in Abbotsford Place. In the first month of operation Dr. Harris did ninety-one consultations on the premises and saw a further twenty-two patients in their homes. Within a few months the system appeared to be functioning well with an increasing number of cases on the register. However, the wider Jewish community was slow to support the Dispensary financially and the President, Joseph Fox, remarked that:

> This institution ought to be supported by every Jew and Jewess as it is the means of preventing many of our people from going to the missionary dispensaries where, very often, after receiving medicine for the body they get a double dose of poison for the soul.[63]

The Jewish Dispensary also appointed a dentist, A. L. Marco, to provide free dental treatment, regularly filling, dressing and extracting teeth of over 50 patients. The popularity of the Fund gradually increased. No less than £121, about half the projected budget, was collected in penny subscriptions in 1913, representing a membership of over 500. In addition to the subscriptions of the poor, additional subventions came from the Glasgow Jewish Board of Guardians and charitable collections at weddings and circumcisions.[64] Concern about the medical missionary societies continued even after the establishment of the Jewish Dispensary, and the newly established Glasgow Jewish Representative Council was asked to circularise the community on the issue in 1914.[65] The Council issued a warning to Jewish parents not to let their children attend the mission halls to collect medicines, as there was a Jewish Dispensary available.[66]

Saul Harris served as medical officer to the Jewish Dispensary until he was called up for military service in 1916, and his place was taken for a short time by Solomon Bridge, son of the Rev. Isaac Bridge, formerly the minister at the South Portland Synagogue. Dr.Isaac Harry Lipetz, who was then given the post, dealing regularly with 500 consultations and house calls anually, succeeded him.[67] The Jewish Dispensary continued to function into the 1930s when the emphasis was on maternal and child health and preventive medicine.

The conflict and competition between the Jewish welfare services and the Christian missionaries continued for many years after the First World War. Some Christians looked on the Jewish discomfort at missionary activities as the price the Jews should be expected to pay for living in a Christian country.[68] Yet it was not just the Jews who saw fault in the whole missionary enterprise. Christian critics pointed to the harm they believed that the missionary effort produced. Charles Booth, pointing to 'professional converts wander(ing) in search of the temporal benefits of Christianity', considered that it 'produces an atmosphere of meanness and hypocrisy and brings discredit both to charity and religion'.[69]

In the final analysis, Glasgow Jewry undoubtedly benefited from the additional services supported by their community as an alternative to missionary provision. Thus, one of the fears of the missionaries, that they would strengthen the Jewish community, actually came to pass. The missionaries had few new members to show for their decades of effort but the Jewish community felt that they had emerged from the encounter stronger, more self-reliant and confident of the support of the Church leadership in the key political and welfare issues of the day.

References

1 Todd M Endelman, *Jewish Apostasy in the Modern World* (New York, 1987), p.1.
2 Kenneth Collins, *Second City Jewry: the Jews of Glasgow in the Age of Expansion 1790–1919* (Glasgow, 1990), pp.44,72.
3 Christopher Clark, *The Politics of Conversion: Missionary Protestantism and the Jews in Prussia 1728–1941* (Oxford, 1995), p.109.
4 Don Chambers, 'Prelude to the last things: the Church of Scotland's mission to the Jews', *Records of Scottish Church History Society*, Vol. XIX, 1975, p.57.
5 *Ibid.*, p.43.
6 Nigel Cameron, editor, *Dictionary of Scottish Church History and Theology* (Edinburgh, 1993), pp.83,84,262,263,275,745.
7 *Glasgow Herald*, 13/1/1909.
8 Fred Levison, *Christian and Jew: the Life of Leon Levison 1881–1936* (Edinburgh, 1989), pp.67–68.
9 *Ibid.*, p.33.
10 David Daiches, *Was: A Pastime from Time Past* (London, 1975), p.36.
11 *Glasgow Post Office Directory*, 1900–1901, p.290.
12 *Jewish Chronicle*, 4/1/1924.
13 Christopher Clark, *op.cit.*, p.186.
14 *Church of Scotland Women's Association for the Christian Education of Jewesses*, 58th Report, 1904, p.13.
15 Anon., *One Hundred Years of Witness* (Glasgow, 1993), p.102.
16 *Glasgow Herald*, 23/11/1906.
17 Fred Levison, *op.cit.*, p.148.
18 Christopher Clark, *op.cit.*, p.275.
19 Fred Levison, *op. cit.*, p.28.
20 *Jewish Chronicle*, 14/4/1891.
21 *Jewish Chronicle*, 28/10/1892.
22 *Glasgow Post Office Directory*, 1900–1901, p.154.
23 *Jewish Chronicle*, 8/12/1905.
24 *Jewish Chronicle*, 7/8/1908.
25 Fred Levison, *op.cit.*, Chapter 14, 'Disputatious Rabbi', pp.144–159.
26 *Ibid.*, pp.147–148.
27 Fred Levison, *op.cit.*, pp.83–84; letter from Otto Schiff, Hon. Secretary, Fund for the Relief of Jewish Victims of the War in Russia, *Jewish Chronicle*, 4/2/1916.
28 *Jewish Chronicle*, 24/8/1919.

29 *Ibid.*, p.151.
30 Kenneth Collins, *op.cit.*, p.87.
31 *Jewish Chronicle*, 9/2/1894.
32 *Jewish Chronicle*, 23/2/1894.
33 *Jewish Chronicle*, 16/3/1894.
34 *Jewish Chronicle*, 13/4/1894.
35 *Jewish Chronicle*, 15/5/1896.
36 *Post Office Directory*, 1894–5; Kenneth Collins, *op.cit.*, p.64.
37 *Post Office Directory*, 1901, p.205.
38 *Post Office Directory*, 1908, p.1721.
39 Kenneth Collins, *op.cit.*, p.103.
40 *Post Office Directory*, 1901, p.205.
41 *Jewish Chronicle*, 5/10/1900.
42 *Jewish Chronicle*, 5/1/1900.
43 *Jewish Chronicle*, 12/11/1900.
44 *Jewish Chronicle*, 24/2/1911.
45 Arnold White, *The Destitute Alien* (London, 1892), p.176.
46 *Glasgow Herald*, 23/11/1906.
47 David McDougall, *In Search of Israel: A Chronicle of the Jewish Missions of the Church of Scotland* (London, 1941), pp.120–121.
48 Records of Glasgow Presbytery, 2/10/1895, CH2/171/27/2, Mitchell Library.
49 *Missionary Record of the United Free Church of Scotland*, 1902, Vol.2, p.126.
50 David McDougall, *op.cit.*, p.121.
51 *Jewish Chronicle*, 22/9/1916.
52 *Jewish Chronicle*, 3/8/1917.
53 G Black, Health and Medical Care of the Jewish Poor of the East End of London 1880–1939, unpublished PhD thesis, University of Leicester, 1987, p.172.
54 Lara Marks, *Model Mothers: Jewish Mothers and Maternity Provision in East London 1870–1939* (Oxford, 1994) p.249.
55 House Committee Minutes, Victoria Infirmary, 24/10/1908, 6/4/1909, GGHB Archives, Mitchell Library.
56 *Jewish Chronicle*, 9/9/1910.
57 *Jewish Chronicle*, 27/1/1911.
58 *Jewish Chronicle*, 17/2/1911.
59 *Jewish Chronicle*, 17/2/1911.
60 *Jewish Chronicle*, 24/2/1911.
61 *Jewish Chronicle*, 21/4/1911.
62 *Jewish Chronicle*, 1/3/1912.
63 *Jewish Chronicle*, 28/3/1913.
64 *Jewish Chronicle*, 29/5/1914.
65 Kenneth Collins, *op.cit.*, p.188.
66 *Jewish Chronicle*, 2/6/1916.
67 Fred Levison, *op.cit.*, p.145.
68 Charles Booth, *Life and Labour in London* (London, 1892), Vol.3, p.177.
69 *Ibid.*, Vol.7, pp.277–8.

Conclusion

'A maximum of reasonable persistency and a minimum of fuss.'
Bailie Michael Simons explaining Glasgow Jewry's favoured method of dealing with the wider community, *Jewish Chronicle*, 24/3/1911

The story of Jewish integration in Glasgow, and the community struggle for health, is a story that was repeated in other communities in Western Europe and North America. Jewish immigrants naturally looked to their more established co-religionists for assistance, and usually help was forthcoming. If the Garnethill, or any comparable leadership elsewhere, had any thoughts that there was any alternative to aiding their weary and impoverished brethren, the public clamour over such issues as sweated labour and alien immigration ensured that the settled communities had to take action.[1]

That action included the provision of welfare facilities supplemented by a range of self-help services initiated by the immigrants themselves. The newcomers increasingly established their own institutions to complement those based at Garnethill. It was perhaps inevitable that there was some tension in the institutional relationships between those who had arrived in Glasgow before the main wave of immigration in the 1890s, and the later arrivals. We have seen that the disbursement of charity was often fairly heavy-handed, in keeping with the ways of the time, and this in itself was a stimulus to self-help. Jews were proud of their ability to care 'for their own', keep Jews out of the Poorhouse and accelerate Jewish integration that would make the newcomers seem less 'foreign'. While the welfare state was in a rudimentary state during this period of immigration, there was enough statutory provision to ease some of the financial burdens that could otherwise have been intolerable.

The Jewish struggle for health had a number of different strands. There was the need to provide medical, welfare and social services for the poor and sick. Jews had to ensure that their co-religionists were able to benefit from statutory welfare and health provision and that they were not discriminated against in the hospitals and other institutions. In particular, they vigorously opposed Christian attempts to exploit Jewish poverty and suffering for missionary purposes. For the children of the Jewish immigrants there was the prospect of following in the chain of Jewish tradition, and the footsteps of Asher Asher by qualifying in medicine.

Thus, the Jewish response to the health and welfare challenges in the immigrant period owed much to the situation and opportunities of the time. While Jewish charitable traditions formed an essential part of the ethos of the community, Jews were more likely to be spurred to action by the plight of their co-religionists and the need to be seen, both by city and non-Jewish neighbours, to be acting decisively. As Liedtke has shown in his studies of Hamburg and Manchester, Jewish provision did not just match what was on offer in the wider community. It was more extensive in quality and quantity than available elsewhere and it provided Jews with the opportunity to strengthen their Jewish identity.[2] In an increasingly secular society Jews turned to Jewish health and welfare groups as a means of helping to retain their Jewishness in a socially accepted form.

Glasgow, and its Jews, frequently point to an absence of anti-Semitism in the city. While, on the whole, there was little overt anti-Jewish prejudice during the period of settlement, it cannot be said that there was no discrimination. The housing market was one particularly sensitive area. There were instances of harsh attitudes in a number of different sectors. There was the denial of Jewish religious needs, such as kosher food in the hospitals or Sunday trading. Evidence of anti-Semitic attitudes could be seen in the psychiatric case-records, and most Jews saw the Christian attempts to convert them as a crude form of anti-Semitism, as it questioned the legitimacy of their religion.

In the years after the First World War the Jewish community built on their earlier achievements, enhancing their new institutions and enriching the life of the city while still preserving much of what made the Jewish community different, culturally and religiously. We have seen that the Jewish community liked to keep a low profile and its institutions preferred to act with a 'maximum of reasonable persistency and a minimum of fuss' even it was slow in achieving results.[3] The Jewish community considered that one of its main tasks was to reduce asssimilation and retain Jewish distinctiveness. Jewish social and welfare societies aided the Jewish community in supporting the sick and needy but provided a framework in which Jews could work and interact together. As Liedtke observed, Jews used these facilities to promote their integration into the wider society, yet these same facilities were important in ensuring continuing Jewish separateness.[4]

Thus the Glasgow Jewish struggle for health maintained two clear components. One part involved making use of statutory provision, sometimes supplementing what was on offer with specifically Jewish input, such as kosher food. The other emphasised the strengthening of Jewish welfare bodies, making them sensitive to the religious and ethnic needs of the Jewish community. Glasgow Jewry was enabled to create a society that ensured its survival as a vital part of local civic and national Jewish life.

References

1 David Vital, *A People Apart: the Jews in Europe 1789–1939* (Oxford, 1999), pp.330–331.
2 Rainer Liedtke, *Jewish Welfare in Hamburg and Manchester c1850–1914* (Oxford, 1998), pp.232–234.
3 'Glasgow's Foremost Jew: an interview with Michael Simons', *Jewish Chronicle*, 24/3/1911.
4 Rainer Liedtke, *op.cit.*, p.234.

Bibliography

Newspapers, Periodicals and Yearbooks

British Medical Journal
Glasgow Herald
Glasgow Post Office Directories, 1890–1914
Jewish Chronicle
Jewish Echo, Glasgow
Jewish Year Book, 1896–
The Lancet
North British Daily Mail
Post Office Directories, 1880–1920
The Times
Yiddishe Vanen Tsaitung, Glasgow

Government and Church Papers

Aliens Act (1905), *Annual Report 1908*, Parliamentary Papers, Cd4102, Vol.87
Aliens Act (1905), *First Annual Report 1907*, Parliamentary Papers, Cd3473
Annual Report of the Church of Scotland Women's Association for the Christian Education of Jewesses, 1904
Census of Scotland for 1891, Gorbals District, Register House, Edinburgh
Minutes of the Glasgow Presbytery of the Church of Scotland, 1890–1914, CH2/171/27/2, Glasgow City Archives, Mitchell Library
Mission Records of the United Free Church of Scotland, 1900–1910, Mitchell Library
Records of Scottish Bankruptcies, National Archives of Scotland, Edinburgh
Royal Commission on Alien Immigration, 1903
Sessional Papers of the House of Lords, Session 1889, Vol.VIII
Records of Bankrupts in Scotland, 1850–1910, National Archives of Scotland
Report of the Interdepartmental Committee on Physical Deterioration, PP 1904, Vol. XXXII

Local Government Papers

First Annual Report of the Committee of the Cemetery to the Merchants' House, Glasgow, 1835, Mitchell Library, Glasgow
Glasgow Municipal Commission on Housing for the Poor (Glasgow, 1904), in Glasgow City Archives (Mitchell Library)
Gorbals Public School Log 1890–1900, Glasgow City Archives, Mitchell Library, Glasgow
Report of the Medical Officer of Health of Glasgow 1908, p.150, DTC 7/11/3, Glasgow City Archives, Mitchell Library, Glasgow

Reports of the Glasgow Sanitary Department 1906–1914, Glasgow City Archives, Mitchell Library
G S Wilson, Memorandum by the Medical Officer of Health on the Presence of Trachoma in Certain Alien Immigrants, in Report of the Medical Officer of Health for Glasgow (1905), pp.130–131, file DTC 7/11/3, Glasgow City Archives, Mitchell Library, Glasgow

Health Records

At GGHB Archives, Mitchell Library unless otherwise noted

Glasgow Ophthalmic Institution, *Annual Report 1907*
Glasgow Eye Infirmary Minutes, GGHB 3/1/4, p.351a
Minutes of the West Cadder Parochial Medical Board, 1858–1862
Patient Case Records 1890–1920, Govan Parochial Asylum and Govan District Asylum
House Committee Minutes 1908–1909, Victoria Infirmary, Glasgow
Patient Case Records 1890–1910, Crichton Royal Infirmary, Dumfries

Jewish Records

SCOTTISH JEWISH ARCHIVES CENTRE, GARNETHILL SYNAGOGUE
Annual Reports, Glasgow Jewish Board of Guardians, 1912–1916
Recollections of Jack Cowen, Gertrude Jacobson Orphanage, 24/9/1995
Letter, from Arthur and Company, Queen Street, Glasgow to Michael Simon, Hon. Secretary, Glasgow Hebrew Congregation, 13/10/1875, Glasgow Hebrew Congregation Letters Book
Letters Book of the Glasgow Hebrew Congregation, 1858–1880
Minutes of the Glasgow Hebrew Congregation, 1858–1919
Minutes of the Glasgow Hebrew Philanthropic Society, 1875–1881
Minutes of the Garnethill Hebrew Congregation
Minutes and Records of the United Synagogue of Glasgow, 1898–1906
Register of Births, Marriages and Deaths, Glasgow Hebrew Congregation
Register of Burials in the Jewish Cemeteries in Scotland

LONDON METROPOLITAN ARCHIVES, 40 NORTHAMPTON ROAD, LONDON EC1
Minutes of the Visitation Committee of the United Synagogue, 1885
Minutes of the Executive Committee of the United Synagogue, 1870–1902
Minute Book of the United Synagogue Council, Vol.1, 1870–1879

HARTLEY LIBRARY, UNIVERSITY OF SOUTHAMPTON
Annual Reports of the London Jewish Board of Guardians, 1862–1866
Minutes of Medical Committee of the London Jewish Board of Guardians, 1873
London Jewish Board of Guardians Subcommittee on Medical Relief, 1861
Minutes of the Executive Committee of the London Jewish Board of Guardians, 1866–1874
Notes and Correspondence of Asher Asher, including letters from Chief Rabbi Nathan Adler

University Theses (unpublished)

Ben Braber, Integration of Jewish Immigrants in Glasgow 1880–1939, University of Glasgow PhD, 1992

Gerry Black, Health and Medical Care of the Jewish Poor in the East End of London: 1880–1939, PhD, University of Leicester, 1987

Rabbinic Literature

Mishna, *Shabbat* 19,2

Babylonian Talmud, *Shabbat* 133b

Shir HaShirim Rabbah, I,15,1

Moses Maimonides, *Yad Milah*, 2,2

Articles and Papers

Jonathan Andrews, A failure to flourish? David Yellowlees and the Glasgow School of Psychiatry: Part 1, *History of Psychiatry*, viii, 1997, pp.177–212

Jonathan Andrews, A failure to flourish? David Yellowlees and the Glasgow School of Psychiatry: Part 2, *History of Psychiatry*, viii, 1997, pp.333–360

Jonathan Andrews, Case Notes, Case Histories, and the Patient's Experience of Insanity at Gartnavel Royal Asylum, Glasgow, in the Nineteenth Century, *Social History of Medicine*, Vol.11, pp.255–282

C C Aronsfeld, German Jews in Dundee, *Jewish Chronicle*, 20/11/1953

Stanley M Aronson, Trachoma and Immigration, *Medicine and Health*, Rhode Island, Vol.80, March 1997

Albert Benjamin, The Old Concept of Jewish Welfare, *Jewish Echo*, 27/5/1988

Stephanie Blackden, The Poor Law and Health: A Survey of Parochial Medical Aid in Glasgow, 1845–1900, in T C Smout, ed., *The Search for Wealth and Stability, Essays in Economic and Social History presented to M W Flinn* (London, 1979)

Geoffrey D.M. Block, Jewish Students at the Universities of Great Britain and Ireland – excluding London 1936–1939, *Sociological Review*, 34, 1942

J Boldt, *Trachoma*, trans. J H Parsons and T Snowball (London, 1904)

James Brown, An Account of the Jews in Glasgow City 11/9/1858, *The Religious Denominations of Glasgow*, Volume 1 (Glasgow 1860)

P S Brown, Herbalists and Medical Botanists in Mid-Nineteenth Century Britain with Special Reference to Bristol, *Medical History*, 1982, Vol.26, pp.407–440

Linda Bryder, A Health Resort for Consumptives: Tuberculosis and Immigration to New Zealand, 1880–1914, *Medical History*, 1996, Vol.40, pp.453–471

Don Chambers, Prelude to the Last Things: the Church of Scotland's mission to the Jews, *Records of the Scottish Church History Society*, 1975,Vol.XIX, part 1, pp.43–58

E Treacher Collins, Introduction, in J Boldt, *Trachoma*, trans. J H Parsons and T Snowball (London, 1904)

Kenneth Collins, Asher Asher MD (1837–1889), Doctor of the Poor, *Glasgow Medicine,* 2, 1984, pp.12–14

Kenneth Collins, Orthodoxy and Reform: Differing Practices in a Glasgow

Jewish Victorian Family, *Korot: the Israel Journal of the History of Medicine and Science*, Vol.11, 1995, pp.54–65

Stephen D Corrsin, Aspects of Population Change and of Acculturation in Jewish Warsaw at the end of the Nineteenth Century: the Censuses of 1882 and 1897, in Wladyslaw T Bartoszewski, Anthony Polonsky, eds., *The Jews in Warsaw: A History* (Oxford, 1991), pp.212–231

M Anne Crowther, Poverty, Health and Welfare, in W Hamish Fraser and R J Morris, eds., *People and Society in Scotland*, Volume II, 1830–1914 (Edinburgh, 1990)

Deborah Dwork, Health Conditions of Immigrant Jews on the Lower East Side of New York: 1880–1914, *Medical History*, Vol.25, 1981

W M Feldman, Tuberculosis and the Jew, *The Tuberculosis Year Book*, Vol.1, 1913–1914

Rona Gaffney, Poor Law Hospitals: 1845–1914, in Olive Checkland and Margaret Lamb, eds., *Health Care as Social History: the Glasgow Case* (Aberdeen, 1982)

L Grassic Gibbon and Hugh Macdiarmid, Glasgow, *Scottish Scene* (1934)

Anne Hardy, Urban famine or urban crisis? Typhus in the Victorian city, in R.J. Morris and Richard Rodger, eds., *The Victorian City: A Reader in British Urban History 1820–1914* (London, 1993)

Anne Hardy, Cholera, quarantine and the English preventive system 1850–1895, *Medical History*, Vol. 37 (1993), pp.250–269

Bernard Harris, AntiAlienism, Health and Social reform in Late Victorian and Edwardian Britain, *Patterns of Prejudice*, Vol.31, 1997

A Henry, Among the Immigrants, *Scribner's*, March 1901

David Heron, The Influence of Defective Physique and Unfavourable Home Environment on the Intelligence of Schoolchildren, *Eugenics Laboratory Memoirs,* VIII, (Cambridge, 1910), pp.58–59

Margaret Lamb, The Medical Profession, in Olive Checkland and Margaret Lamb, eds., *Health Care as Social History: the Glasgow Case* (Aberdeen, 1982)

Dorothy E Lindsay, *Report upon a study of the Diet of the Labouring Classes in Glasgow: carried out during 1911–1913 under the auspices of the Corporation of the City* (Glasgow, 1913)

I S L Loudon, A Doctor's Cash Book; the economy of general practice in the 1830s, *Medical History*, Vol.27, 1983, pp.265–266

Alexander Macgregor, Physique of Glasgow Children admitted to the City of Glasgow Fever Hospital, Belvedere during the years 1907–1908, *Royal Philosophical Society of Glasgow,* Vol.40, 1908, p.172

J C McDonald, The History of Quarantine in Britain during the 19th Century, *Bulletin of the History of Medicine*, Vol.25, 1951, pp.22–44

Howard Markel, "The Eyes Have it": Trachoma, the Perception of Disease, the United States Public Health Service, and the American Jewish Immigration Experience, 1897–1924, *Bulletin of the History of Medicine*, Vol.74, 2000, pp.525–560

Hilary Marland, The Medical Activities of Mid-Nineteenth Century Chemists and Druggists, with special reference to Wakefield and Huddersfield, *Medical History*, Vol.31, 1987, p.415

Karl Pearson and Margaret Moul, Problem of Alien Immigration into Great Britain: Illustrated by an Examination of Russian and Polish Jewish Children,

Annals of Eugenics, Volume 1, pp. 5–128 (1925–6); Volume 2, pp.111–245 (1927); Volume 3, pp.1–76 and pp.201–262
Report on the Physical Condition of Fourteen Hundred Schoolchildren in the City, City of Edinburgh Charity Organisation Society (London, 1906)
Report of the *Lancet* Special Sanitary Commission on the Sweating System in Glasgow, *Lancet*, 30/6/1888, pp.1313–1314
Report of the *Lancet* Special Sanitary Commission on the Sweating System in Edinburgh, *Lancet*, 23/8/1888, pp.1261–1262
Frank Rice, Care and Treatment of the Mentally Ill, in Olive Checkland and Margaret Lamb, eds., *Health Care as Social History: the Glasgow Case* (Aberdeen, 1982), pp.60–73
Kasim M J Al-Rifai, Trachoma through history, *International Ophthalmology*, Vol.12, 1988, pp.9–14
S Rosenbloom, Jewish Charitable Relief in the Provinces, *Jewish Chronicle*, 14/9/1906, pp.26–27
Theodore B Sachs, Tuberculosis in the Jewish District of Chicago, *JAMA*, Vol.43, 1904, pp.390–395
Thomas Schlich, Medicalisation and Secularisation: the Jewish Ritual Bath as a Problem of Hygiene (Germany 1820s-1840s), *Social History of Medicine*, Vol.8 (1995), pp.423–442
Leonard D Smith, Insanity and Ethnicity: Jews in the Mid-Victorian Lunatic Asylum, *Jewish Culture and History*, Vol.1, 1998, pp.27–40
T S Wilson, The Incidence of Trachoma in Glasgow 1914–1968, *Health Bulletin*, Vol. XXVII, July 1969
Elizabeth Yew, Medical Inspection of Immigrants at Ellis Island 1891–1924, *Bulletin of the New York Academy of Medicine*, Vol.56, June 1980

Books

Anon., *One Hundred Years of Witness* (Glasgow, 1993)
Anon., *The Conversion of the Jews* (Edinburgh, 1842)
Geoffrey Alderman, *The Jewish Community in British Politics* (Oxford, 1983)
Geoffrey Alderman, *Modern British Jewry* (Oxford, 1992)
R D Anderson, *Education and Opportunity in Victorian Scotland* (Oxford, 1983)
Jonathan Andrews, *They're in the Trade . . . of Lunacy, They 'cannot interfere' - they say. The Scottish Lunacy Commissioners and Lunacy Reform in Nineteenth-Century Scotland* (London, 1998)
Asher Asher, *On Circumcision* (London, 1873)
Asher Asher MD 1837–1889: Collected Writings (London, 1916)
Chaim Bermant, *Coming Home* (London, 1976)
Chaim Bermant, *Troubled Eden: An Anatomy of British Jewry* (London, 1969)
Charles Booth, *Life and Labour in London* (London, 1892), Vols. 3, 7
Lilian Brandt, *The Social Aspects of Tuberculosis: based on a study of statistics*, Committee on Tuberculosis, (New York, 1902)
Eugene C Black, The Social Politics of Anglo-Jewry 1880–1920 (Oxford, 1988)
Callum G Brown, *Social History of Religion in Scotland* (London, 1987)
Nigel Cameron, *Dictionary of Scottish Church History and Theology* (Edinburgh, 1993)
A K Chalmers, *The Health of Glasgow 1818–1925: An Outline* (Glasgow, 1930)

A K Chalmers, ed., *Public Health Administration in Glasgow: A Memorial Volume of the Writings of James Burn Russell* (Glasgow, 1905)
Olive Checkland, *Philanthropy in Victorian Scotland: Social Welfare and the Voluntary Principle* (Edinburgh, 1980)
Olive Checkland and Margaret Lamb, eds., *Health Care as Social History: the Glasgow Case* (Aberdeen, 1982)
Christopher Clark, *The Politics of Conversion: Missionary Protestantism and the Jews in Prussia 1728–1941* (Oxford, 1995)
James Cleland, *Enumeration of the Inhabitants of the City of Glasgow and the County of Lanark for the Government Census of 1831* (Glasgow, 1831)
Kenneth E Collins, ed., *Aspects of Scottish Jewry* (Glasgow, 1987),
Kenneth E Collins, *Go and Learn: the international story of the Jews and medicine in Scotland 1739–1945* (Aberdeen, 1988)
Kenneth E Collins, *Second City Jewry: the Jews of Glasgow in the age of Expansion 1790–1919* (Glasgow, 1990)
M Anne Crowther and Brenda White, *On Soul and Conscience: the Medical Expert and Crime* (Aberdeen, 1988)
David Daiches, *Two Worlds* (Sussex, 1971)
David Daiches, *Was: A Pastime from Time Past* (London, 1975)
David Daiches, *Glasgow* (London, 1977)
John Efron, *Defenders of the Race: Jewish Doctors and Race Science in Fin-de-Siècle Europe* (Yale, 1994)
John M Efron, *Medicine and the German Jews: A History* (New Haven, 2001)
Todd M Endelman, ed., *Jewish Apostasy in the Modern World* (New York, 1987)
David Feldman, *Englishmen and Jews: Social Relations and Political Culture: 1840–1914* (New Haven, 1994)
Peter Fyfe, *Backlands and their Inhabitants* (Glasgow, 1901)
John A Garrard, *The English and Immigration 1880–1910* (London, 1971)
Lloyd P Gartner, *The Jewish Immigrant in England 1870–1914* (London, 1973)
Sander Gilman, *Franz Kafka, the Jewish Patient* (New York, 1995)
Sander L Gilman, *Freud, Race and Gender* (Princeton, 1993)
Sander L Gilman, *The Jew's Body* (New York, 1991)
Sander L Gilman, *Smart Jews: the Construction of the Image of Jewish Superior Intelligence* (Lincoln, 1996)
Sander L Gilman, *Love + Marriage = Death, and other Essays on Representing the Difference* (Stanford, 1998)
Ralph Glasser, *Growing up in the Gorbals* (London, 1986)
Ralph Glasser, *Gorbals Boy at Oxford* (London, 1988)
Gerald N Grob, *Mental Illness and American Society 1875–1940* (Princeton, 1983)
David Hamilton, *The Healers: A History of Medicine in Scotland* (Edinburgh, 1981)
Anne Hardy, *The Epidemic Streets: Infectious Disease and the Rise of Preventive Medicine 1856–1900* (Oxford, 1993)
Colin Holmes, *Anti-Semitism in British Society 1876–1939*, (London, 1979)
Bernard Homa, *Metzitza* (London, 1966)
Irving Howe I with Kenneth Libo, *The Immigrant Jews of New York: 1881 to the present* (London, 1976)
Ronald Hyam, *Empire and Sexuality: the British Experience* (Manchester, 1990)
Louis Hyman, *The Jews of Ireland: from Earliest Times to the Year 1910* (Shannon, 1972)

Louis Jacobs, *Theology in the Responsa* (London, 1975)
Immanuel Jakobovits, *Jewish Medical Ethics* (New York, 1967)
Jewish Encyclopaedia (New York, 1925)
Jacob Katz, *Divine Law in Human Hands: Case Studies in Halakhic Flexibility* (Jerusalem, 1998)
David Kohn-Zedek, *Bet Asher* (Hebrew), bound with *Asher Asher MD 1837–1889: Collected Writings* (London, 1916)
Fred Levison, *Christian and Jew: the Life of Leon Levison 1881–1936* (Edinburgh, 1990)
A. Levy, *Origins of Glasgow Jewry 1812–1895* (Glasgow, 1949)
Rainer Liedtke, *Jewish Welfare In Hamburg and Manchester c1850–1914* (Oxford, 1998)
Roland Littlewood, Maurice Lipsedge, *Aliens and Alienists: Ethnic Minorities and Psychiatry*, 2nd edition (London, 1993)
David McDougall, *In Search of Israel: A Chronicle of the Jewish Missions of the Church of Scotland* (London, 1941)
Alexander Macgregor, *Public Health in Glasgow: 1905–1946* (Edinburgh, 1967)
Howard Markel, *Quarantine! East European Jewish Immigrants and the New York City Epidemics of 1892* (Baltimore, 1997)
Lara Marks, *Model Mothers: Jewish Mothers and Maternity Provision in East London 1870–1939* (Oxford, 1994)
Hilary Marland, *Medicine and Society in Wakefield 1780–1870* (Cambridge, 1987)
C H May and C Worth, *A Manual of Diseases of the Eye*, revised M L Hine, 9th edition (London, 1946)
Charles Newman, *The Evolution of Medical Education in the Nineteenth Century* (London, 1957)
Sir John H Parsons, *Diseases of the Eye*, revised H B Stallard, 10th edition (London, 1947)
M. Jeanne Petersen, *The Medical Profession in Mid-Victorian England* (London, 1978)
Julius Preuss, *Biblical and Talmud Medicine*, trans. Fred Rosner (New York, 1978)
Edna Robertson, *Glasgow's Doctor, James Burn Russell 1837–1904* (East Linton, 1998)
Cecil Roth, *The Rise of Provincial Jewry: the Early History of the Jewish Communities in the English Countryside 1740–1840* (London, 1950),
Mordechai Rozin, *The Rich and the Poor: Jewish Philanthropy and Social Control in Nineteenth Century London* (Brighton, 1999)
James A Schmiechen, *Sweated Industries and Sweated Labour: The London Clothing Trades 1860–1914* (London, 1984)
Emmanuel Shinwell, *Conflict Without Malice* (London, 1955)
R. Shlomo Zalman Sonnenfeld, *Guardian of Jerusalem: The Life and Times of Rabbi Yosef Chaim Sonnenfeld*, adapted by R. Hillel Danziger (New York, 1983)
Michael E Teller, *The Tuberculosis Movement: A Public Health Campaign in the Progressive Era* (New York, 1988)
Samuel Thomson, *New Guide to Health* (Columbus, Ohio, 1827)
Angela Tuckett, *The Scottish Trades Union Congress: the First 80 Years* (Edinburgh, 1986)

David Vital, *A People Apart: the Jews of Europe 1789–1939* (Oxford, 1999)
Michael R Weisser, *A Brotherhood of Memory: Jewish Landsmanshaftn in the New World* (New York, 1985)
Arnold White, *The Destitute Alien* (London, 1892)
Bill Williams, *The Making of Manchester Jewry 1740–1875* (Manchester, 1985),
Charles Winston, *Lodge Montefiore No.753: 1888–1988* (Glasgow, 1988)
Charles W J Withers, *Urban Highlanders: Highland-Lowland Migration and Urban Gaelic Culture 1700–1900* (East Linton, 1998)
Frank Worsdall, *The Tenement, A Way of Life: A Social, Historical and Architectural Study of Housing in Glasgow* (Edinburgh, 1979)

Glossary of Hebrew and Yiddish Words

Beth din: Jewish law court. It usually deals with matters of *kashrut*, that is regulations pertaining to kosher food, or to personal matters, e.g. in registering of marriages and arranging divorces.

Bikur cholim: visiting the sick, often used to refer to a society organised for sick visiting on a regular basis.

Brit milah: circumcision of baby boys, carried out at 8 days old.

Chevra: brotherhood or society, often organised for prayer.

Cheder: lit. room; Hebrew and Jewish religious education classes usually held after school or on Sunday morning.

Chovevei Zion: lit. lovers of Zion; early Zionist society. The first Glasgow branch was founded in 1891.

Chupa: lit. wedding canopy; the Jewish marriage ceremony.

Der heim: lit. the home; the Jewish areas left behind by the immigrants in Eastern Europe.

Di goldene medine: lit. the golden land, usually referring to America where the streets were believed to be 'paved with gold'.

Fusgayers: young Jewish walkers who trekked across Europe from Rumania to Britain in 1899.

Get (pl. *gittin*): Jewish religious divorce.

Halacha: lit. the way; the authoritative code of Jewish law.

Kaddish: prayer of praise to God recited during synagogue services and by mourners during the year after the death of a parent and on the anniversary of a death (*yahrzeit*).

Kosher: food prepared in accordance with Jewish religious laws, especially of *shechita* (qv) and keeping meat and milk foods separately.

Landsleit: persons from the same area of Eastern Europe.

Landsman: person from the same area of Eastern Europe (plural: *landsleit*)

Landmanschaft: society linking immigrants from the same East European town or *shtetl (*qv).

Mikva: ritual bath used by married women for law of 'family purity'.

Minyan: prayer quorum of ten males above the age of religious responsibility at *bar mitzvah* (13 years).

Mohel: skilled religious official, who does not have to be a doctor, who carries out the ritual of *brit mila*, circumcision.

Rabbi: teacher and spiritual leader of the Jewish community.

Rav: preferred rabbinic title of many orthodox rabbis.

Shechita: Jewish method for despatch of animals for food, carried out by a trained *shochet* (qv).

Shiva: week of intense mourning after the death of a close relative.

Shochet: highly skilled religious official who carries out the rapid and painless killing of animals for food according to the Jewish laws of *shechita* (qv).

Shtetl: village in Eastern Europe, often overwhelmingly Jewish in population.
Shul: synagogue.
Shulchan Aruch: compendium of Jewish law covering every aspect of Jewish life.
Talmud Torah: organisation providing elementary Jewish education.
Treifa: usually refers to food that is not religiously fit for Jewish consumption.
Yiddishkeit: observance of Jewish religion and culture.
Yom Kippur: Day of Atonement. Solemn fast day of prayer and penitence; the holiest day in the Jewish year.

Index